LIVING WITH ITCH

A Johns Hopkins Press Health Book

Living with

Itch

A Patient's Guide

Gil Yosipovitch, M.D., and
Shawn G. Kwatra, M.D.

The Johns Hopkins University Press
Baltimore

© 2013 The Johns Hopkins University Press
All rights reserved. Published 2013
Printed in the United States of America on acid-free paper
9 8 7 6 5 4 3 2 1

The Johns Hopkins University Press
2715 North Charles Street
Baltimore, Maryland 21218-4363
www.press.jhu.edu

Library of Congress Cataloging-in-Publication Data

Yosipovitch, Gil.
    Living with itch : a patient's guide / Gil Yosipovitch, M.D., and
Shawn G. Kwatra, M.D.
        pages cm.—(A Johns Hopkins Press health book)
    Includes index.
    ISBN 978-1-4214-1233-7 (pbk. : alk. paper)—ISBN 1-4214-1233-0 (pbk.
: alk. paper)—ISBN 978-1-4214-1234-4 (electronic)—ISBN 1-4214-1234-9
(electronic)—ISBN 978-1-4214-1235-1 (interactive book)—ISBN 1-4214-
1235-7 (interactive book)
    1. Itching—Popular works. 2. Skin—Diseases—Popular works. 3. Der-
matology—Popular works. I. Kwatra, Shawn G., 1986- II. Title.
    RL721.Y67 2013
    616.5—dc23   2013016433

A catalog record for this book is available from the British Library.

*Special discounts are available for bulk purchases of this book. For more infor-
mation, please contact Special Sales at 410-516-6936 or specialsales@press.jhu
.edu.*

The Johns Hopkins University Press uses environmentally friendly book
materials, including recycled text paper that is composed of at least 30
percent post-consumer waste, whenever possible.

The facing page is a continuation of this copyright page.

We would like to thank Josh Tan for sharing his expertise and for traveling to help make this book possible.

We would like to thank William Safrit, Carrie O'Sullivan, and Anne Marie Johnson for their technical assistance.

We would like to thank Julie Block and the Coalition of Skin Diseases for their tremendous help with this book project.

We would like to thank Eric Kageyama, Krista Kellogg, Kaspar Mossman, and Susan Thornton for sharing their stories.

GY: I gratefully dedicate this book to all of those patients who suffer from chronic itch and continue to teach me daily lessons about this disease and its impact on their quality of life. I also dedicate this book to my loving wife, Galit, children, Natalie and Dan, and my parents, Shifra and Zvi, for their support, patience, and love.

SK: I dedicate this book to my devoted parents, Madan and Neelam, and sister, Gita, for their constant encouragement, love, and support.

CONTENTS

PART III. TREATING ITCH

FOREWORD

Until the mid-1990s, itch was a neglected subject. There had been very little research on it, and there was no treatment for itch as good as aspirin is for pain. Indeed, some drugs that relieve pain actually *cause* itch. (Doctors also use the term *pruritus* when talking about itch. The terms are interchangeable.)

Gil Yosipovitch became interested in the basic science and clinical aspects of itch around that time. Before long, he had founded the International Forum for the Study of Itch (IFSI) and become its first president. In 2013, IFSI held its Seventh World Congress on Itch.

Dr. Yosipovitch is driven to study itch. His research has greatly enhanced our understanding of itch and furthered our ability to treat it.

This book and its inventive format will make it possible for people who suffer from itch to understand it more completely. And its practical advice will help *everyone*—from anyone who has ever been bitten by a mosquito to anyone who has ever experienced the unrelenting itch of the many skin diseases in which it causes so much suffering.

JEFFREY D. BERNHARD, M.D.
Professor Emeritus of Dermatology, University of Massachusetts Medical School
Editor Emeritus, *Journal of the American Academy of Dermatology*

Chronic itch is a problem affecting millions of people worldwide. The goal of this book, available in both print and interactive formats, is to provide people with the information they need to better understand and manage their conditions. We start with the basics of itch and then provide an overview of the mechanisms responsible for itch transmission. After this, emphasis is placed on specific itchy conditions and unique types of itch. Last, we wrap up with a discussion of the various forms of treatment.

One of the aspects of this book that we are especially proud of is the emphasis on the emotional and psychological aspects of itch. With this in mind, the book includes several interviews and essays from people suffering from chronic itch.

We hope that this book will help provide all people (patients and doctors) with a better appreciation of chronic itch and inspire them with hope as they march forward.

Terms in **bold** are defined in the glossary. "Did you know?" features are cued with the symbol ▣. Also, throughout this book, you will see symbols for videos ▶ and interactive graphics ▚. Visit the associated website links for multimedia features on chronic itch.

A Patient's Perspective
Eczema: A Lifelong Conflict

It's not every day that you see your photo in the *New York Times*.

Actually the *Times* has never run my photo, but on July 1, 2003, a series of images in the science section captured one aspect of my life so perfectly that I might as well have been the subject. Three frames from a video, featuring a Japanese man, asleep, but far from at peace—writhing in torment as he scratches his chest, his arms, his back.

The accompanying story described the studies of Gil Yosipovitch, a professor of dermatology at Wake Forest University in Winston-Salem, North Carolina, and an expert in chronic itch.

I've suffered from chronic itch all my life: forty years and counting. I have eczema. A dermatologist told me I was the worst case she'd ever seen. Genetics and environment may have combined to intensify my condition. My paternal grandfather, a legendary curmudgeon, had eczema, and it afflicts my sister, my daughter, and a cousin. I spent my first decade on the Canadian prairie, with its extremely dry and hot summers and bitter winters. And my father smoked cigarettes in the house until I was seven years old.

 See jhupress.com/livingwithitch/ for a video interview with Kaspar M., who has atopic dermatitis (eczema).

Whatever the causes, I've spent countless nights in the grip of itch, tearing at my skin to wake in the morning with crusty gashes on my hands, face, and elsewhere. As I type these words, under the stress of composing prose, I reach under my desk to scratch the back of my knees. To live with eczema is to fight a war for control of your own body—with the goal of enjoying life, even temporarily, as people with normal skin do.

Adult eczema, like many chronic diseases, resembles a conflict in one of the world's many trouble zones. Cyprus, the Balkans, east Africa, Palestine: a bomb explodes, crowds riot, soldiers shoot, things calm down, diplomats talk, but nothing ever gets resolved.

Eczema flares are one aspect of the conflict. Sometimes there's an obvious cause: I am terribly allergic to cats, but I enter the house of a friend who owns one. Or I eat something that contains cayenne pepper, a vicious trigger. Sometimes there is no apparent reason. Still, after a few days or weeks, my skin clears. The episode is a battle of sorts. I would like to think that in some cases I win, when I exert control. I identify the trigger and prevent myself from exposure: stay away from cats; eat a bland diet. I employ my arsenal of topical steroids. I smear on thick moisturizing cream. I practice yoga to relax.

Beyond flares, the broader conflict with eczema takes place on many fronts. Most of the time, nobody knows that you are fighting but you. Nobody cares but you. But when you win, the triumph is all yours.

Self-control in Public

Most people associate eczema with childhood. And children are not expected to control themselves, so nobody blames them when they scratch. An adult who scratches, by contrast, seems immature. Not many people understand how itchy someone with eczema can feel and how it can be impossible to restrain yourself from scratching. Even my own father, when I was twenty-two, told me that adults don't scratch and it was time to grow up. (And his father had eczema!)

Even when you're not scratching, the scars of your previous

bouts with eczema disfigure your hands and face. As you ride the subway, order in a café, or make a PowerPoint presentation at work, eyes are judging you.

Unfortunately it's not easy to stop scratching. Most of the time it's not even an option. Some of the worst episodes of scratching come at night, when I am asleep, and I literally have no control. During the day, I sometimes experience intense episodes of itch brought on by stress or other triggers, which only a life-or-death threat can override.

However, you *can* cure yourself of a certain kind of scratching that most people would class as a bad habit. I indulge in this type of scratching to relieve nervous energy or when I'm bored. I discovered on the Internet several varieties of psychological training that you can do by yourself or with a professional to quit. I tried one, "habit reversal," after learning about it from Christopher Bridgett, a psychiatrist in London.

In habit reversal, first you make yourself aware of how much you scratch. Then you intercept each impulse, and clench your hands instead, or perhaps dig your nails into your palms to create a bit of pain to mask the itch. Over time, you feel less inclination to scratch. Habit reversal worked for me. Maybe my brain now associates the sensation of itch with the punishment of pain instead of the reward of scratching. Your training can lapse, so you must keep it up.

Sleep

Although my sleep is mostly peaceful these days, for much of my earlier life (if you'll permit a slight exaggeration) my nights resembled the film *A Nightmare on Elm Street*, in which Freddy Krueger roams the dreamscape with blades for fingernails. Except I was both Freddy and victim.

I went to a coed boarding school in the UK, starting at the age of thirteen. For the first four years, I slept in a dormitory with ten to fourteen other boys. In my third year, a friend informed me that the previous night, he'd heard a strange sound and looked across to see me tearing at my head in a frenzy. This was the first time I realized what my hands were doing at night. I became increasingly aware that once I fell asleep, I lost control. My hands ran amok, leaving painful scratches for me to deal with the next day.

In my fourth year, I decided to show my hands who was boss. Once lights were out, I bound my hands with rope, locking the ends together with a padlock. I hid the key under my pillow. Unfortunately, I chafed my wrists bloody against the rope. But I continued to bind my hands at night.

Eventually, this resulted in a social disaster. In the fifth year I got my own room. After an evening spent boozing at the local pub—we were of legal age, and seniors were officially allowed to have two drinks—I turned in for the night. For some reason, a classmate came in and switched the light on to wake me up. He saw that my hands were tied; assumed someone else had played a prank on me and called in a posse to witness me shackled to the bed, woozy and incoherent. Because I had drunk so much, I didn't even remember the episode until someone mentioned it at breakfast the next day. Then I realized the fever dream was real. For the rest of the year, people looked at me oddly.

My skin didn't improve at university, mostly because I insisted on staying up late several nights a week, drinking at pubs and bars where everyone smoked. I majored in physics. I don't know whether it would have been different if I'd chosen English, as I found my weekly problem sets incredibly stressful. Night after night I'd wake up scratching furiously, half-dreaming that by attacking the itch, I was solving some mathematical puzzle. I often found my face torn up in the mornings. I wore cotton gloves, but that only meant that I rubbed my skin raw instead of scratching it. Doctors prescribed antihistamine pills that did nothing.

I never won the sleep battle. But eczema doesn't affect my sleep at the moment. So what happened?

I think it's because my lifestyle and environment changed. I grew up, and no longer need or want to party late or have more than one drink, if any. I'm done with school: no more tests and homework anxiety. Almost everywhere, laws have made it illegal to smoke in public places, so I'm no longer exposed to irritating cigarette smoke. I live in a temperate climate, where the air isn't dry or humid. And I'm married, and my wife stabilizes me emotionally. (We have young kids, who cause us all kinds of grief, but I love them, so things even out.) My eczema has mellowed with time.

It's worth pointing out that I drank, hung out with smokers, and studied physics by choice. If I hadn't done those things, my eczema might have been less severe. But this perspective is clear only in hindsight. At the time, I just didn't realize it. I was finding my own way.

Bullies

Let's go back to that morning after the night when my schoolmates found me tied to my bed. There I was at breakfast, and the awful realization dawned that everyone who mattered in my social life now knew that I suffer from eczema so badly that I handcuffed myself to stop scratching. I was horribly embarrassed.

Eczema will do that to you. And the teenage years are such an intense period in your self-definition and social development that I wouldn't be surprised if most adults with eczema said that high school was their worst period. Eczema's out there on your skin where everyone can see it. Insecure people looking to deflect attention from their own defects can point at you. And the injustice! You feel bad enough already, and people are singling you out for abuse. The casual, biting comments can burn for a lifetime.

Here's the remark I remember more than any other, twenty-two years later. It was the last year of high school. I was having an eczema flare, part of which peeked out, red and angry, above my collar. Maybe the room was full of people, maybe it wasn't—all I remember is the other boy, and his words.

"What's been chewing on your neck?"

I wanted to evaporate. I remember making some reply. Then I holed up in my room until nightfall.

I can't ask for sympathy. In high school, I made similar comments to other boys and girls that they probably still remember, about their looks or weight or accent or so on. But I'd like to ask what you can do when someone says something mean to you.

Some of us are gifted with wit and can turn an insult back at the one who spoke it or spin it into a joke. I don't have that gift. But I do remember what people said to shut me up when I teased or harassed them: "Why are you such a bastard to me?"

I had no answer (though, in truth, it would have been "because I'm insecure"). So I stopped immediately. The direct approach can work.

As can other tactics, like rolling with the punches. At the end of senior year I found myself at a table in the cafeteria, with some girls and a boy who was eager to score points with them. He asked loudly whether I remembered the time they had all found me tied to the bed because I was so crazy with itch. Inside I shriveled with shame, but I nodded, grinned, and laughed as if I had found it as funny as he had. He pushed as far as he could, but I endured until by persisting he risked embarrassing himself. He had to change the subject.

Fortunately high school doesn't last forever. We graduate, and as we mature we realize that everyone is carrying a burden, some physical or mental problem that they would wish away if they could. Migraines, depression, back pain. We have enough troubles of our own, so we go easier on those around us.

God help you if you teach high school, though.

Allergies

My eczema has never been a problem for my romantic partners, despite my teenage fears. (It certainly doesn't make you any more confident with the opposite sex, though.) A former girlfriend told me, during an angst-filled breakup, that "it was never about your skin." Apparently I have other flaws!

I took the aftermath of that breakup as an opportunity to tackle a long-postponed challenge: to search, with as much rigor as possible, for the foods that I was convinced were triggers for my eczema. Since I lived and grocery shopped alone, I was able to cut out whole food groups for weeks at a time and see what made a difference. The results surprised me.

I had read that the major food allergens are found in dairy, soy, wheat, nuts, and fish; also, I had identified other suspects such as tomatoes and citrus. I quit drinking coffee. I threw out the contents of my spice cabinet and, for a draconian half-year, stopped eating at restaurants because I couldn't be sure what the cooks were putting in the food.

After two weeks of a diet of little more than oatmeal, rice, lamb, and a small list of vegetables and fruit, I was amazed to find that my skin had almost completely cleared up. I could actually see blue veins on the back of my hands, which had previously burned red with eczema. I reveled in my new freedom to take my shirt off while hiking on hot days.

Then I began adding foods back in, two weeks at a time. Wheat. Soy. Dairy. Tomatoes. Oranges. Not a single whole food turned the eczema back on again.

What I did notice, though, was that alcohol—particularly spirits and certain wines—caused problems, as did hot spices. My conclusion was that alcohol and spices make your skin hot and flushed, and somehow the increased blood flow makes you itchy, even hours afterward.

The rice vinegar in sushi was also deadly. A few years later I thought I would explore fine cheeses and, after one of the most unbearable nights of my life, realized that aged cheese contained a mystery essence of itch. That essence, I learned from Internet searches, was histamine, a component of many aged and fermented foods such as pickles. Red wines, especially burgundies, contain a lot of histamine, which is probably why they make me feel itchy.

I also had a skin prick allergy test done, which revealed that I was likely allergic to cats, which I was well aware of; rye grass pollen, which made clear that my environment might be a factor; and egg white, which explained why I itched like a flea-bitten dog after drinking eggnog every Christmas. The allergy test wasn't particularly helpful by itself, but it contributed to a growing sense that I was understanding my disease and gaining a degree of control over it.

Infection

If you have eczema, you learn to live with the threat of infection. My own worst scare came when I was sixteen and had found that I could quell my itchy scalp by pulling out small clumps of hair. I thought this was a fine discovery. But after a few days, little fluid-filled blisters started creeping over my torso. They spread to my face—and everywhere. I looked like a medieval plague victim.

We were in Germany at the time (my father, a professor, was on sabbatical near Frankfurt) and my mother took me to the dermatologist. Language was not much of a barrier. He prescribed two strengths of cream which he said were "very powerful." Fortunately, the medication cleared up the rash, which I realized later must have been eczema herpeticum.

Several times since then I have had widespread *Staphylococcus aureus* infections. The first time I had one, it was because I had just started using a super-strong steroid ointment and had applied it over too much of my skin at once. Amoxicillin cleared that outbreak up, but I kept the vial of antibiotic capsules and proceeded to self-medicate with them, one or two at a time, every few weeks or so. That was colossally stupid, because the next staph infection I had didn't respond to amoxicillin. I had created a resistant strain. (Dicloxacillin killed that one off.)

What I've learned about infections and eczema is this: be aware of the first signs of infection, and respect your antibiotics. Complete the course of medication properly, and throw away any pills you have left over. If you monkey with your meds, you only create trouble.

Travel

Eczema has made me less spontaneous throughout my life than I might have been without it. When I was in college, I couldn't just crash at someone else's house, or go on a road trip, unless I wanted to be dry, itchy, and inflamed the next day. I have never enjoyed traveling, because it takes me far from my stock of ointments and therapies at home and guarantees that I'll have to scour the shelves of a strange pharmacy for fragrance-free soaps and creams. If a staph infection flares up, I won't be able to get antibiotics. In a lot of situations—a youth hostel, for example—I won't have the privacy to apply moisturizer properly. Then I suffer later.

When I do travel, at some point my enjoyment of the trip is likely to be overshadowed by eczema. Maybe food will play a role, but general stress (particularly that of air travel and its schedules, connections, delays, and security hassles) is almost guaranteed to trigger a flare. Then, it doesn't matter where I might be—Havana, Rome, Salt Lake City—my focus turns inward, rather than outward. Instead of enjoying the exotic culture or architecture or ski slopes, I hunker down into endurance mode, thinking of my return, when I can shower, use tar shampoo, moisturize and apply steroids, and hide in my own house away from the eyes of others.

My loss, you may say. Why can't I ignore temporary discomfort and salt away some brilliant memories? But that's the way it is.

However, itch exists only in the present tense. I can never remember how itchy I was in the past. My memories, if I were able to ignore eczema, would be exactly the same as those of a "normal" person. That goes for a weekend, a school term, or my entire life. If I had been able to ignore eczema, I wouldn't realize now that I had been itchy then. But because of eczema, I have fewer pleasant memories than you might. That is a shame.

And so, if I had a recommendation, it would be to get out and travel as much as you can. Bring your personal pharmacy with you. Do all you can do, and try to put the trials of eczema out of your mind. In the future, you will thank yourself for it.

Parenthood

Becoming a father put eczema in a new perspective for me. My five-year-old son does not have eczema; I am grateful. My three-year-old daughter does—but not as severely as I do, for which I am also grateful. Having children, and passing on a disease such as eczema that has a strong genetic component, makes me aware of my temporary place in my greater family's unfolding story. The genes I passed on were as much mine as they were my parents', and my grandparents', and so on.

I do feel guilty to some degree that I "gave" my daughter the disease, but it's not like I chose which genes went into her DNA. The consolation is that I can bring my experience to bear. I know the proper way to moisturize her skin and the difference between a slight outbreak and a dangerous flare or infection that needs a doctor's appointment.

Being a father helps me understand my own parents. They did not have eczema themselves, so had no idea how to deal with it. Doctors weren't that much help. That is why I didn't find out about real moisturizers or steroids until I was an adult.

I feel curiously detached when I watch my daughter scratch. Of course I'm sympathetic, because she's my daughter and she's clearly in torment. However, my first instinct is to tell her to stop scratching, which I know is completely useless. Now I understand how my parents must have felt and how my wife feels when she sees me scratching.

Eczema is predominantly a childhood disease, so I can hope— even though adult eczema is widespread in my family—that one day soon my daughter might be free of symptoms. Probably she will not, though, and then I will have to watch from the sidelines as she fights all her own battles. It will be hard for me, but perhaps she will find her own way to succeed.

There is no getting around the fact that eczema does not come with much of a silver lining. It is true that you are one of the lucky few who know the ecstasy of a good scratch, but eczema makes your life worse in many ways. You fight your battles, and the best you're aiming for is to have a normal day like everyone else.

But when I get depressed, I keep in mind that as bad as I might feel, I have much to be thankful for: a good education, a loving family, a satisfying job. There are people who wish they had my problems. There is a phone book's worth of debilitating or terminal diseases that I don't have. And neither do my children, who can look forward to living normal lives. What more could I ask for?

PART I

Definitions and Mechanisms of Itch

1
What Is Itch?

What Is Itch?

Be it a mosquito bite, contact with poison ivy, or the consequence of one of many chronic diseases, all of us have experienced itch at some point in our lives. What is itch? One excellent definition comes from the German dermatologist Samuel Hafenreffer, who first defined itch in 1660 as an "unpleasant sensation provoking the desire to scratch." It is important to define the differences between acute and chronic forms of itch.

Acute Itch

Acute itch is a sensation that causes the urge to scratch for a limited time. This time period can range from only a few seconds to up to six weeks. This form of itch is typically located in a specific area and can be caused by local trauma such as a reaction to an insect bite. Whatever the cause, acute itch features localized

 Did you know?

"Pruritus" (a Latin term) is a technical word doctors often use for "itch."

Did you know?

Chronic itch has cognitive, emotional, medical, and sensory components and can severely affect quality of life, often leading to depression, anxiety, severe sleep problems, or thoughts of suicide.

inflammation (swelling) that can usually be successfully treated by common therapies such as antihistamines and corticosteroids.

Chronic Itch

Chronic itch is defined as lasting for longer than six weeks. A key difference between acute and chronic itch is that chronic itch usually originates from within the body. Indeed, chronic itch can be a sign of complex medical problems such as dermatologic and systemic diseases. A systemic disease affects a number of organs in the body or the entire body. Other causes of chronic itch include long-term exposure to external agents such as poison ivy or nickel.

Treatments that are effective for acute itch may not relieve chronic itch, because they are not directed toward the underlying cause. Thus, itch relief for people suffering from chronic itch (if attainable) is temporary and will return promptly when therapy is discontinued.

Chronic itch that cannot be treated is known as *intractable itch*. Many people with intractable itch have tried numerous therapies that failed to provide relief. The cause of itch in these people cannot be removed; sometimes the cause remains unknown.

Epidemiology: How Many People Have Itch?

Itch is the principal symptom of most skin disease and is associated with many systemic conditions (such as liver disease, renal failure, hematologic abnormalities, and endocrine disorders). Although we don't know how many people have itch, some studies give us an idea of what percentage of the population suffers with itch. A large Norwegian study found the prevalence of itch to be approximately 8% in adults. A recent study of more than 11,000 German workers showed the incidence rate of chronic itch to be 17%. This study also revealed that itch prevalence increased with age and that approximately 25% of people with itch suffered from itch for more than five years. Estimated itch prevalence rates for selected dermatologic and systemic diseases are displayed in tables 1.1 and 1.2.

Table 1.1. Estimated itch prevalence rate for selected skin disorders

Dermatologic condition	Prevalence rate (%)
Atopic dermatitis	100
Scabies	100
Urticaria (hives)	97
Extensive psoriasis	80
Burns	67–87
Acne	50
Dry skin associated with old age	30–60

Table 1.2. Estimated itch prevalence rate for selected systemic diseases

Systemic causes	Prevalence rate (%)
Hyperthyroidism	60
Anorexia nervosa	58
Polycythemia vera	48
Hodgkin's lymphoma	30
Chronic renal failure (on hemodialysis)	25–85
Chronic liver disease	20–25
Diabetes	11
Hepatitis C	4

2

What Causes Itch?

Anatomy of Itch

The skin is composed of an upper layer known as the *epidermis* and a lower layer called the *dermis* (figure 2.1). Itch emanates from the upper layers (the epidermis and the junction between the epidermis and dermis, called the *epidermal/dermal transition*). Indeed, while your muscles, joints, and internal organs can be painful, they do not itch, because itch is transmitted only from the upper layers of the skin.

Neural Transmission of Itch

The skin features a dense network of nerves that convey itch signals from the skin to the brain. Starting in the skin, a major mode of communication of itch signals is through *C nerve fibers*, a subset of nerve fibers that have a very slow conduction speed

Did you know?

A study more than fifty years ago demonstrated that people who have the upper layers of the skin removed can still feel pain but not itch.

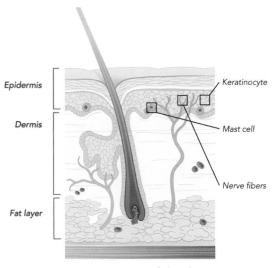

Figure 2.1 Parts of the skin.

Epidermis

Dermis

Fat layer

Keratinocyte

Mast cell

Nerve fibers

(only 2 to 8 cm/second). Once C fibers in the skin detect an itchy sensation, this impulse travels to an area close to the spinal cord known as the *dorsal root ganglion*. From the dorsal root ganglion, these neurons cross sides and ascend upward toward the brain following a tract referred to as the *lateral spinothalamic tract*. The lateral spinothalamic tract ends at a part of the brain called the thalamus, which projects messages about an itchy stimulus to a number of different brain areas that are involved in the sensory, cognitive, and emotional aspects of itch and scratch.

See jhupress.com/livingwithitch/ for an interactive graphic on the itch pathway from the skin to the brain.

 ## Did you know?

The *lateral spinothalamic tract* is a bundle of sensory nerves that ascends from the spinal cord to the brain. In addition to transmitting itch signals, it also carries sensory information about pain and temperature sensations.

Specific Itch Pathways

The above-mentioned C nerve fibers that carry itch messages from the skin to the brain can be further classified into two categories: *histamine sensitive* and *non-histaminergic*.

Itch triggered by histamines

Histamine is an important chemical that is released from **mast cells** in the skin. Mast cells are a part of the immune system. Inside them are tiny granules containing different chemicals that cause inflammation and itch such as histamine and **proteases**. When mast cells release histamine, an inflammatory response is activated. Examples of histamine-sensitive itch transmission include itch associated with hives as well with as other signs of inflammation, such as insect bite reactions and drug rashes.

Itch not caused by histamines

Since most forms of itch are not triggered by histamines, we say they follow a *non-histaminergic pathway*. Examples include itch of eczema and psoriasis and itch of systemic diseases, such as uremic itch.

Itch Transmission

The upper layer of the skin, spinal cord, and brain are all involved in itch transmission. At each of these levels, messages containing itch signals are transmitted through many microscopic **mediators**, or chemicals, that bind to their corresponding **receptor** in the skin or nervous system. A group of receptors on the cell membrane that share similarities in their structure are named *G-protein coupled receptors*. Examples of these receptors that have been shown to be involved in the transmission of itch include the following: proteinase activating receptor, **neurokinin** 1 receptor, and gastrin-releasing peptide receptor.

In addition to G-protein coupled receptors, some receptors work on **ion channels**, referred to as the *Transient Receptor Potential (TRP) ion channel family*. Some TRPs have thermal sensors (a way to think of this is like a microscopic thermometer) that can modulate various stimuli, such as itch; this could be an explanation for why application of an ice cube or other cooling agents, such as menthol, reduce itch. Other TRP channels are activated by spices, such as capsaicin, and compounds like camphor that have been used for centuries in China and are highly involved in itch transmission.

 See jhupress.com/livingwithitch/ for an interactive graphic on itch receptors.

The specific involvement of some of these receptors in disease states (which will be discussed in more detail later; for example, see chapter 7) is displayed in table 2.1.

Similarities with Pain

Itch and pain share many similarities. Both of these conditions are bothersome symptoms that follow the same neural pathway, traveling through the nervous system via the lateral spinothalamic tract (as detailed above). However, when you encounter something that is painful, such as accidentally touching a hot stove, your response is to withdraw your hand. Conversely, an itchy stimulus leads directly to a scratching reflex. When people scratch such a bothersome area, itch sensation is reduced because of the pain induced by scratching. Painful stimuli have also been

Table 2.1. Itch mediators and associated skin diseases

Mediator/Receptor	Type of receptor	Major associated skin diseases
Histamine / Histamine receptor	G-protein coupled	Urticaria
Proteinases / Proteinase activating receptors (PARs)	G-protein coupled	Atopic dermatitis, acne
Substance P / Neurokinin 1 receptor (NK1R)	G-protein coupled	Atopic dermatitis, cutaneous T-cell lymphoma, psoriasis
Transient Receptor Potential (TRP) channels	Thermal	Neuropathic itch, psoriasis
Opioids / Opioid receptors	G-protein coupled	Uremic pruritus, cholestatic pruritus
IL-31 / IL-31 receptor	Cytokine	Atopic dermatitis, cutaneous T-cell lymphoma

shown to inhibit itch experimentally, using chemical, electrical, mechanical, and thermal stimuli. In fact, many common itch therapies, such as very hot or cold showers, inhibit itch in this way.

There are also many similarities between chronic itch and constant pain. One such similarity is that nerve fibers are overactivated in both conditions, which cause stimuli to be perceived as increasingly itchy or painful (a condition referred to as *hypersensitization*). In people suffering from chronic itch, painful stimuli such as an electric shock may be interpreted as itch. Similarly, in people who suffer from chronic pain, an itchy stimulus may lead to the aggravation of pain.

Did you know?

Pain and itch can have an inverse relationship. If pain is induced, itch is inhibited. Is the reverse true? Well sometimes when pain is inhibited, people will itch. An example of this is when people take pain medications, such as morphine—pain is reduced but people can start to itch!

PART II

Different Forms of Itch

A Parent's Perspective
An Unexpected Life

I've been coming to this spot on the shores of Lake Tahoe for more than thirty years. Time and change have moved swiftly, walking hand-in-hand. I have a son now, Jarrett, who is seven years old. He is already growing beyond the age for me to carry him. He and his younger sister, Shay, have become adept at climbing over these same shoreline rocks as I once did, splashing in the same majestic waters. As the sun reveals itself over the horizon, I look out over the endless blue of the sky. In shorts, a sleeveless shirt, and flip-flops and listening to nothing but the water gently touching the shore, I think back on the decade that just passed. A morning boater passes by, disturbing the stillness and sending small waves crashing against the rocky shoreline. The water gradually calms, continuing again like an old man in his rocking chair, breathing steadily. People see life through eyeglasses forged specifically for them. My prescription has changed many times through the years and will continue to do so until my last breath, I suppose. I can honestly say, this is not the life I had imagined for myself.

 See jhupress.com/livingwithitch/ for a video interview with Eric K., the father of a child who has atopic dermatitis (eczema).

The first time I recall hearing of eczema was as a teenager. I had a crush on a girl from a neighboring school. She had flowing black hair just below her shoulders and a face I couldn't wait to lay my eyes on. As we got to know one another I noticed that the skin from just below her ear to the base of her neck was red, dry, and flaking. She had this way of holding her hair over that area of her neck, but she must have seen my eyes attempting to decipher the flakes and patches that would occasionally peek out from behind those tresses. She finally told me one day it was something called eczema. I did not know what eczema was, and, never having been exposed to the disease, I was afraid to touch her skin. As much as I crushed on this young beauty, I eventually distanced myself. Years later, I would hear that she went on to a successful career in the medical field. Some two decades after that, the disease I once ran away from would find its way back into my life and inexorably change its course.

At thirty-two years of age, I was living the American dream. I had just gotten married; purchased a newly built, three-story home; had a bright financial future; and my first child was on the way. But that optimism would soon face an unimaginable storm. Three months after Jarrett was born the redness began to appear on the skin of his creases—his elbows and knees. Initially we tried to explain it away, not realizing it was the beginnings of a disease that may challenge Jarrett for, perhaps, the rest of his life. He was a chubby child, so I thought the rash was a result of chafing. But over the next couple of months it spread over his entire body and attacked his skin in the form of open sores and lesions. He would claw into himself, lashing back at the skin that mercilessly and relentlessly attacked him. At the end of these flare-ups, large chunks of his skin were left looking like raw meat, cracking and oozing with pus and blood. The eczema overwhelmed Jarrett's body. He would receive shocked and sympathetic looks from friends and strangers alike, so much so, I often felt the need to reassure people that it was not contagious. And yet they seemed to keep their distance, leaving us, his parents, feeling that they were passing judgment.

When the pediatrician first diagnosed Jarrett with atopic

dermatitis (eczema), our reaction was: "It's a struggle, but he'll grow out of it." She prescribed a steroid cream and referred us to an allergist so Jarrett could be tested in hopes of revealing the cause. We completely relied and trusted what the pediatrician was telling us. Who were we to question? We were so desperate; we followed the advice of and dispensed medication prescribed by anyone who had an office and an M.D. on their door: apply a steroid cream and moisturize with a bath followed by over-the-counter lotions and creams. We were given no assurances. There was an almost continuous, 24/7 palpability to the tension in our home. We had no answers or cure for this vicious malady that had taken over Jarrett's life. We were not about to leave the care of our ailing son to a day-care provider or nanny. Fortunately, Jarrett's mother was able to stay home with him. I would leave for work at 6 a.m. and would often return home after 6 p.m. I called her cell phone several times a day to check on Jarrett, wanting to be with him at every moment.

When it came time to go to the allergist, I took off work to be there. I did not expect the world to stop because I had my problems to deal with at home, but I was surprised at the conflicting guilt I felt when it came to taking time off from the family business because of Jarrett's doctors' appointments. The silence from others did not mask their judgments. When we took Jarrett to the allergist, he was still much too young to verbally articulate his emotions. However, the pleading in his expressions ripped away at my spirit. There would be two visits to the allergist's office. During the first visit, Jarrett had only a small patch on his back that was clear enough to do the prick tests. I held Jarrett as the nurse navigated her pen around the inflamed areas, creating a map-like configuration for the test to be applied. I recall having a strong hope that this test would pinpoint which types of food were triggering these massive reactions with his skin. That once we figured out what was causing this he would be fine within days. When it came time to apply the test, I held both of Jarrett's wrists while his mother held his legs steadily. He screamed in agony as I tried in vain to calm him. My wife was sobbing. I could literally feel his small wrists swelling within my grip. My fortitude betrayed me. I told the nurse to stop the test. Nothing felt right about what we were doing. My wife convinced me to continue, saying that we were already there and this would eventually help us find out what was causing his eczema. I closed my eyes as tears rolled down my cheeks. We continued the test.

The second visit proved to be much like the first. The results: allergies to tree nuts, peanuts, soy, dairy, shellfish, dust mites, eggs, and few other things I cannot recall. Now we were of the mind that virtually any food had the possibility of causing a reaction. Jarrett's diet was completely broken down. Until he was nearly four years old, his entire food intake was of plain chicken, broccoli, and a small portion of white rice. No breads, fish, cereals, beef, milk, and not a lick of sweets or cakes that other kids his age took for granted.

My sister, whose daughter suffers from extremely severe allergies and eczema, warned me about the dangers of steroid medication and regulating food intake, so I had several preconceived notions regarding how we should handle Jarrett's eczema. While I would continuously ask her for advice, she made it very clear that we had to find our own path in helping Jarrett. A lotion, cream, therapy, or method that works for one often fails for another. At the time, I didn't understand what she meant or how accurate her words were.

The pediatrician visits and trips to the allergist left us with more questions than answers. I remember feeling more like a naïve patron waiting at the traveling medicine cart, given remedies and prescriptions that may hold hidden dangers while acting as only minimally effective salves.

Once Jarrett outgrew wearing mittens, regularly cutting and filing his fingernails every few days became a necessity to lessen some of the damage to his skin and to help prevent him from getting fungal infections beneath his fingernails from all the scratching. This was always a laborious task. I would pin down both of his arms and lightly lay my body over his to keep him from struggling. Eventually, I became immune to his screams. It was not long after our visits to the allergist's office that I had him immobilized on our bed, cutting his nails. His skin was an absolute mess: red, weeping with pus in some areas, and so thick and deeply dry in others, gauze and bandages covering his open wounds. I remember looking into his eyes, trying to read what they were saying. It was at that moment, without provocation, that the skin on his cheek cracked wide open, splitting as if he'd been gashed by a knife's blade. His screams rose to a pitch that left me gasping so deeply I could not catch my breath. Up until that moment I felt as if I had done everything I could for Jarrett but, in hindsight, I had the luxury of leaving for work each day. I at least got some reprieve from having to deal hands-on with the minute-to-minute care Jarrett needed at that time. His mother had none. I cannot imagine what the experiences of seeing her child in a constant state of jeopardy must have done to her. It was at that moment when I knew things had to change.

It wasn't until a friend put us in touch with one of the leading pediatric allergists in Los Angeles that I really felt a health care professional took the time to explain to us just what this atopic dermatitis was that Jarrett's pediatrician had diagnosed him with. We spent close to an hour in his office. He joked with and amused Jarrett while examining his rash-covered body. After the examination he took us to an area where Jarrett played with some toys as the doctor sat with my wife and me on a small couch. He was frank in telling us that we had a very rough road ahead and that there was no magic remedy to make it all go away. He went through the misconceptions and realities of topical steroid use on children. While I had hoped to walk away with that nonexistent therapy or medicine that would cure Jarrett, I was bolstered by the idea that topical steroids, when used properly, were not the horrible poison some had led us to believe. That being said, we are continuously balancing the long-term safety of the medications with the most important thing: the quality of Jarrett's daily life. The doctor went on to recommend some household changes to help neutralize the dust mites, as well as telling us to continue with some of the things that we had already been doing.

We tore out the carpeting on the entire top level of our three-story home and replaced it with bamboo flooring. Vacuuming the remaining carpet and surface cleaning became my daily routine after work. To the detriment of my marriage, each night I would sing John Denver songs to Jarrett to soothe and help him sleep. I would hold his arms to prevent him from scratching while hanging my body over the crib rail, struggling to stay awake. While the rest of the world slept, I continuously prayed for some kind of support, anything. Emotional pain and I became closely acquainted. It left me continuously questioning who planned this pathetic beginning to Jarrett's life. What had this world done to itself that a child, my boy, would have to suffer like this? Was this some sort of punishment that my son had to bear for my past sins? The nights were endless, and the heartache slowly emptied me of who I once was. When Jarrett would appear to fall into a deep sleep, I would tiptoe toward his bedroom door, only to hit a creaky floor board and wake him. The routine repeated itself countless times during the night. The exhaustion, coupled with working a full day on just a few scattered hours of sleep, was too much. With regularity I would doze off on my commute home, many times missing my off ramp on the highway. Eventually, I would take short naps in my car, across the street from my home, before going inside and resuming my routine.

Of course, there were the infinite unsolicited recommendations from the well-intentioned: Emu oil, shea butter, coconut oil, sea salts, countless over-the-counter products, Eastern medicine, homeopathy. Nothing produced any viable results. One went as far as to hand me a bottle of cream she claimed had cured her grandson. It was a product I had never heard of, had no FDA approval, and had a strong medicinal smell. There is always an underlying desperation to find a product that is effective at keeping the itch at bay. I was grateful that she was concerned enough about Jarrett to offer the product but did not give one thought to trying it on him. I learned early on not to fall prey to the Internet advertisers who are often the equivalent of park bench lawyers, preying on the guilt and desperation of the victims of eczema. Our reality was a daily balancing act where advised methods and rules were often not followed. No one told us to do things like take Jarrett to Disneyland in his footie pajamas that covered him from his neck to his feet, with medical tape wrapped around his wrists so he couldn't pull up his sleeves to scratch. Then there were the wrist restraints we used and modified to use in his car seat so he couldn't reach himself to scratch. As we came to rely on giving him antihistamine during incessant and uncontrollable fits of scratching the fear of giving him too much would have to wait for later. For better or worse, we made it up as we went along.

As guarded and vigilant as I am with Jarrett's care, there are always loopholes. Times I know Jarrett may possibly have a reaction to something but choose to be willfully ignorant. Jarrett loves pets and going to other peoples' houses. A good percentage of the time if a residence has a dog or carpeting, Jarrett ends up reacting and scratching uncontrollably. It often comes to a point where we have to leave. It's been a few years now, but I took Jarrett to our local pier to enjoy some father-son time and to have a small snack. I bought a lemonade for us to share and a basket of French fries. This simple pleasure that any child should be able to enjoy ended with a trip to the emergency room. I hadn't realized that the oil they cooked the fries in was probably the same one they used to fry various types of seafood. Jarrett's face ballooned to where he was unrecognizable and caused his eczema to rage out of control. Luckily, there was no anaphylaxis. Now, I cannot go a day without wondering what possible dangers—food or environmental—are out there just waiting to challenge Jarrett.

When the discussion became serious that we wanted a second child, I had two main concerns. One was Jarrett well enough that caring for his eczema and allergies would not hinder our attention toward a second child? And, two, was our marriage strong enough to support another child? Our divided thoughts on the treatment of Jarrett's eczema were a huge concern for me. It had been a tremendous test of the fortitude of our relationship. To that point, I felt we had a vast disconnect. After all, it's hard to be on the same page when each is holding a different book. As things go, Shay was born not long after Jarrett's second birthday. Shay is absolutely gorgeous and quite the character. More important, thus far she has been eczema and allergy free. I have speculated as to why she was spared the affliction that affects Jarrett every moment of his life. The only difference I came up with was that Shay was immediately breastfed at birth, and, though his mother tried to do the same for him in the beginning, Jarrett was quickly formula fed. In the continuous struggle for explanations, she probably just came up favorably in the roll of the genetic dice.

After more than two years of Jarrett's same nighttime routine I relented and brought him to sleep with me in my bed. I would like to say I did so reluctantly, but Jarrett was three years old by that time, and I did not see any real improvement in his skin or sleeping patterns. Though we had since eschewed the footies for shorts and a t-shirt to keep his body temperature cool and his itchiness at bay, he would still wake up to bouts of scratching and was not getting close to the amount of sleep a boy his age should get. By that time, Jarrett's mother had already taken to sleeping downstairs. Any disturbance, any slight movement in the bed, would wake her. So whether it was my snoring, continuously going back and forth to help Jarrett, or other reasons, at some point her bed became the living room couch. It seems we had grown apart, and our marriage—our relationship—had deteriorated to that of roommates.

At a very early age, Jarrett showed a penchant for numbers and memorization. So when I brought home a program from a Los Angeles Lakers basketball game, it was no surprise (and quite delightful for me) that he immediately scanned through it and memorized the players' names and jersey numbers. It soon became a game of sorts where I would ask him questions about the players, and he would point them out on the television screen when they were playing. This proved to be a tremendous part of his nighttime ritual. While I've always tried to develop little games and activities to distract his mind away from scratching, sports—basketball, in particular—became an invaluable tool to keep his mind off the itch. Jarrett would lie beside me and listen intently as I entertained him with bedtime stories of the greatest Laker of them all, Magic Johnson, and how a guy named Michael Jordan made everything seem cool. Now that we were in the same bed, I was able to add hours to my sleep and Jarrett slept better knowing I was by his side. When he did wake up scratching he would often tell me to turn on one of the Lakers' games I had recorded on the DVR. Yes, it was unconventional, but it consistently kept his mind off of scratching. I cannot express the importance of that routine and being able to get the rest we had both so much needed.

I was so focused on Jarrett's care, and now my new baby daughter, I lost sight of much of what was going on around me. With the economy in peril and the bills stacking up, it made financial sense to sell our house. And as life continued to roll on, somewhere along the road my wife and I became emotionally disconnected. I would never put one speck of thought to the idea that Jarrett's eczema was the cause of our marriage failing. I chose to focus solely on Jarrett's care, his eczema and allergies, and my daughter's well-being. That was my choice, period. All else was a distant second. The biggest mistake I made during my marriage, and this journey with eczema, is that I did not take care of myself. The countless nights I lay with Jarrett, praying for a miracle: the therapies, medicines, and cure-alls that proved fruitless.

Eczema is truly a misunderstood disease that seldom goes noticed unless you are affected by it either directly or indirectly. It leaves parents desperate and searching for any shred of hope. As a caregiver dealing with this disease for over seven years now, many of my ideals, beliefs, and loves have changed—or evolved, as I like to believe. Some of the answers an inquisitive Jarrett seeks do not come as easily as they once would have. Hopefully there will be a day when eczema will be a distant memory for Jarrett. For now, I will continue to brush away the dandruff in his hair and wipe away the flakes of skin on his clothing. As life continues to take away his innocence, I hope he will not, one day, question the decisions I made for him in those difficult moments.

This time in my life that I have shared with you has put me on a new path where I really don't know what is going to happen next. But on this new journey I'm learning how to take care of myself and be happy. I have since found a special partner who is committed to helping Jarrett understand his eczema and loves the kids as if they were her own. There truly is such thing as starting over. The other night as I was putting Jarrett to bed, he asked me, "How long am I going to have my eczema?" I thought for a moment and told him, "I don't know Jarrett, but one day it won't be so bad. And then, one day, maybe you can become a doctor and help find a cure for eczema." He grinned a bit and said, "Oh, okay, Dad."

The cool waters of Lake Tahoe washing over the shoreline stop for no one. Where has all the time gone? It's a place my parents used to bring me as a child, and now I bring my own. Jarrett, still dressed in his pajamas and scratching around his neck as he usually does in the morning, has come to join me. Shay and my love are not far behind as they make their way across the sandy beach. The three of them decide to navigate across the same stretch of rocks as I had done for decades. I often wonder what memories Jarrett will carry with him from those dark times, and Shay, for that matter, seeing her brother's continuous struggles with his eczema. The challenges that both of my kids have had to endure at the start of their lives will hopefully propel them as they continue on. Unfortunately, the book of our family's journey with eczema appears several pages from its conclusion. As I lie on the largest, flattest boulder I can find, I motion Jarrett to come to me. I ask him to close his eyes and lie on my chest, his face toward the sky. With all of his weight on me, and lying still as can be, I tell him to open his eyes. He inhales deeply, and I can feel the hope rush through me.

Ours is truly an unexpected life.

3
Atopic Dermatitis

What Is Atopic Dermatitis?

Atopic dermatitis (AD), also known as eczema, is a chronic skin disorder affecting hundreds of millions of people around the world. It has been estimated that 10% of the population will be affected by AD at some point in their lives. AD often follows a waxing and waning course, filled with periods of disease flares and periods of remission. While AD may persist to adulthood, infants and young children are most frequently affected. The hallmark of AD is the terrible itch it causes.

What Causes Atopic Dermatitis?
Role of the immune system

Researchers do not know the precise cause of AD, but evidence points to an involvement of both hereditary and environmental factors. AD is part of an *allergic triad* of conditions that also includes asthma and hay fever (seasonal allergies). These

 Did you know?
"Eczema" comes from a Greek word meaning "to boil over."

conditions are thought to be caused by an inherited predisposition to an overactive immune system. Indeed, substances called **cytokines**, which are secreted by cells in the immune system, are often up-regulated (more numerous) in people who have atopic dermatitis.

Genetic causes

Researchers recently found that patients with atopic dermatitis have a genetic defect in *filaggrin*, a protein that plays a significant role in forming the upper layer of the epidermis, also known as the *stratum corneum*. Without sufficient filaggrin, the skin barrier is weakened and becomes accessible and sensitive to germs, allergens, and many other foreign substances. Since a weakened skin barrier increases nerve fibers' exposure to the environment, people who have atopic dermatitis are more likely to be irritated by exposure to soaps, detergents, and even temperature changes (hot or cold temperatures). Because the skin is missing some of its natural building blocks, many people who have AD suffer the symptoms of dry skin. This is why people who have AD benefit so much from using moisturizers containing **ceramides**, substances that are vital to the barrier of the skin because of their ability to replenish it.

 See jhupress.com/livingwithitch/ for an interactive graphic on how the hypersensitivity of nerve fibers causes itch in atopic dermatitis (eczema).

Skin Manifestations in Atopic Dermatitis

Atopic dermatitis causes significant inflammation and severe itch and scratching, which in combination lead to skin redness

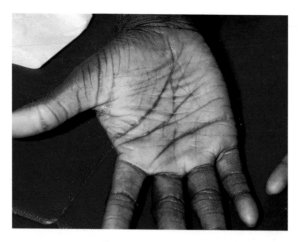

and crusting, scaling, and often oozing skin lesions. These lesions often have a typical distribution in the body, often affecting the skin folds of the arms and behind the knees (figures 3.1 and 3.2) and below the ears (figure 3.3). People from different ethnic groups often have different presentations of atopic dermatitis.

Itch in Atopic Dermatitis

Itch is the primary symptom of people who have atopic dermatitis. Severe and frequent or constant itch leads to many sleepless nights and severely impairs a person's quality of life. Itch in atopic dermatitis is aggravated by proteases, small proteins that are also secreted by *Staphylococcous aureus* (a bacterium that is found in the respiratory tract and on the skin) and house dust mites, common triggers of flares of AD. Scratching is hard to resist and may lead to thickened and darkened areas of skin, bacterial infections, and worsening rashes. AD features a vicious

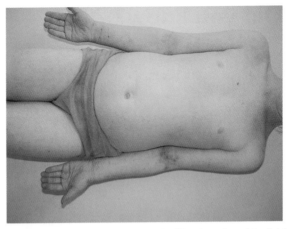

Figure 3.1. Atopic dermatitis (eczema) affecting the skin folds in the forearm of a child. Courtesy of Dr. Elaine C. Siegfried.

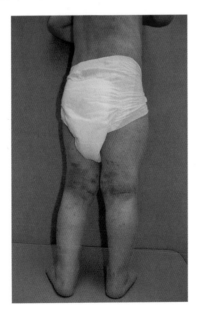

Figure 3.2. Open **erosions** accompanied by lichenification, or thickening of the skin, behind the knees in a child with terrible itch associated with atopic dermatitis (eczema). Courtesy of Dr. Elaine C. Siegfried.

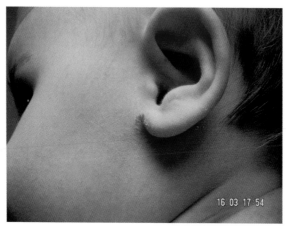

Figure 3.3. A crack in the skin below the earlobe, known as an infra-auricular fissure, often associated with severe atopic dermatitis. Author photo.

itch-scratch cycle. The itch causes you to scratch, and scratching worsens the itch. This cycle keeps repeating itself, leading to damage to the skin barrier as well as breaks in the skin that can lead to infections.

Many people who have atopic dermatitis are not aware of how much they are scratching, particularly during the night, which not only disturbs sleep but further increases skin inflammation.

 See jhupress.com/livingwithitch/ for a video showing a patient scratching at night because of the severity of his itch.

Did you know?

The prevalence of itch in atopic dermatitis may be as high as 100%. Itch is so central to this condition that it has been referred to as "the itch that rashes."

Table 3.1. Common triggers of itch in people who have atopic dermatitis

Environmental factors	Low and high humidity
	Cold and hot weather
	Seasonal allergies
Allergens and irritants	Harsh soaps and detergents
	Food (peanuts and seafood are frequent offenders)
	Pets (cat and dog dander)
	Mite exposure
	Wool
	Perfumes
	Cigarette smoke
Stress	Includes emotional factors such as divorce, loss of a loved one, or other significant life changes
Infections	The most common skin infection is *Staphylococcus aureus*

In addition to interrupting restful sleep, itch in atopic dermatitis can be a contributing factor to psychosocial conditions including depression, anxiety, difficulty concentrating, and poor self-esteem. Similarly, stress is known to be an aggravating factor for itch in people who have atopic dermatitis. Building on this association, a study using brain imaging found that itch in people who have atopic dermatitis significantly differs from itch induced in healthy individuals; that is, itch in people who have AD activated areas of the brain involved in emotion and in the memory of negative experiences. This study highlights the role of cognitive and emotional factors in the exacerbation of itch in AD.

Factors aggravating itch in people who have atopic dermatitis can be broadly categorized as follows: environmental triggers, allergens, emotional stress, and infections. A list of common factors triggering itch in people with AD is displayed in table 3.1.

Treatment of Itch Associated with Atopic Dermatitis

The treatment of itch is specialized based on the age and circumstances of individuals. However, treatment should focus on two fronts: (1) instituting measures for prevention of AD-associated itch and (2) providing symptomatic relief for itch associated with current skin lesions.

Preventing itch

As mentioned above, people who have atopic dermatitis often have a disrupted skin barrier. For this reason it is important to moisturize the skin as soon as possible after bathing, to replenish the skin barrier and prevent water loss and irritation. (Be sure to select a moisturizer that replenishes **ceramide** and other lipids that are depleted in the outer layers of the skin in people with AD.) Indeed, a study found that the amount of water loss in the skin is associated with the intensity of itch. Use low pH cleansers, which are effective at reducing itch because their low pH reduces the activation of nerve fibers that are often overly sensitive to enzymes activated by higher pH cleansers. In addition, patients and their families should try to keep a diary documenting the circumstances surrounding episodes of severe itch and use the diary to try to identify an association between itch or increased itch and specific factors.

Relieving symptoms

Since atopic dermatitis features a hyperactive immune response, drugs that can suppress the immune system (either topically—put on the skin—or systemically—taken orally) are effective in relieving symptoms of itch associated with AD. These drugs are described in table 3.2.

Table 3.2. Classes of medications that can relieve itch associated with atopic dermatitis (AD)

Treatment	Description
TOPICAL TREATMENTS	
Topical corticosteroids	Corticosteroid creams and ointments are anti-inflammatory agents that can be effective in reducing itch. While several over-the-counter corticosteroid creams are available, many doctors prescribe stronger corticosteroid creams. See a list of these creams and more information about topical corticosteroids in chapter 14.
Topical calcineurin inhibitors	Topical calcineurin inhibitors, which are available either as an ointment or a cream, are applied directly to the skin. They include tacrolimus (brand name Protopic) and pimecrolimus (brand name Elidel). These medications are given as prophylaxis and have been proven to be effective in reducing inflammation and itch associated with AD. These agents are particularly useful for the face and armpit regions, areas where topical corticosteroids are traditionally not used due to concern for skin **atrophy**.
Double wet layer pajamas	This therapy usually uses a low- or medium-strength topical corticosteroid that is applied on the skin. The patient wears a double layer of pajamas, featuring a wet inner side and a dry outer side. This therapy is based on occlusion, or increased contact between the topical corticosteroid and the skin. The pajamas should be left in place for approximately 12 hours. This treatment can be repeated once a day for a week. It is particularly effective in people who have severe AD or during acute flares. See chapter 14.
SYSTEMIC TREATMENTS	
Antihistamines	Antihistamines, as their name suggests, work by blocking histamine, which is a potent mediator associated with itch and inflammation. Antihistamines by themselves are not usually able to control itch associated with AD, because other, non-histamine-related pathways are responsible for transmitting itch in AD. It is important to note that most of the effect of antihistamines in AD is through their ability to help people sleep. Please refer to chapter 15 for more detailed information.
Mirtazapine	Mirtazapine is an antidepressant that is particularly effective in relieving itch at night (and in the process halting the vicious itch-scratch cycle).
Systemic corticosteroids	Corticosteroids can be taken orally for a limited time and are typically reserved for severe cases of atopic dermatitis that are unlikely to be resolved by topical treatment alone.

Cyclosporine	Cyclosporine is an oral drug that suppresses the overactive immune system in people who have atopic dermatitis. It should be used if topical and other systemic therapies have not been effective in relieving AD-associated itch. People taking cyclosporine should be monitored closely by their doctor, since it has been associated with some serious side effects including high blood pressure and kidney dysfunction.
Mycophenolate mofetil	Mycophenolate mofetil is a drug that suppresses the immune system. The most common side effects are gastrointestinal symptoms including diarrhea and nausea.
Azathioprine	Azathioprine is a drug that suppresses the immune system. It is often used to treat itch in people who have severe atopic dermatitis. Patients taking azathioprine should have lab work done regularly to check blood counts and liver enzymes.
Methotrexate	Methotrexate is an oral anticancer drug that can be used to suppress the immune system in low doses in people who have AD. It is associated with liver toxicity and should not be taken by women who are pregnant or may become pregnant. Patients should have lab work done regularly to check blood counts and liver enzymes.
Antibiotics	For severe, often oozing infections, antibiotics may be helpful in treating atopic dermatitis lesions and in reducing itch. This is because several bacteria, including Staphylococcus aureus (the most likely offender in AD patients), secrete proteases, small proteins that have been shown to play a role in aggravating itch.
Phototherapy	Phototherapy involves exposing a patient to ultraviolent (UV) light for a specific period. Typically in the treatment of AD, patients may be exposed to different wavelengths of UV light (termed narrowband or broadband). Narrowband UVB light is particularly effective in reducing the itch associated with AD; phototherapy is effective in reducing itch in AD because UV light (at specific wavelengths) is able to modulate the activity of the immune system and decrease inflammation.
Acupuncture	Acupuncture has been shown to significantly reduce itch in people who have atopic dermatitis. However, it should be combined with other therapies.
Psychosocial support	For a person with atopic dermatitis, the treatment can be demanding and requires a coordinated effort from family members. Indeed, parents spend a significant amount of time caring for their kids' skin. AD also has a significant emotional and social effect and can severely disrupt sleep. Physicians can provide education as well as support to help families increase the efficacy of treatment. Indeed, there are several programs that aim to educate families on how to better handle the psychosocial aspects of AD. These "eczema schools" have resulted in better coping skills and treatment for people who have AD.

From Double Helix to Dermis: The Menacing Morse Code of Psoriatic Itch

The itch of psoriasis is like insult to injury; salt to wound; fan to flame. There aren't enough idioms in the world to describe an itch so insidious that it is barely satisfied by uncontrollable, rabid, and mindless self-mutilation. I know that if I scratch at my raw, cracked, and bleeding skin, the resulting carnage will be tender and painful, even more so than it was before. But, there is no choice when it comes to itch like this. This is life with psoriasis. This is life with chronic itch.

The itch of psoriasis is a torment so intense, so unrelenting as to cause a reasonable person to continuously rake her fingernails across the dry, crusty landscapes of skin that are her palms, soles, and tender scalp, much of which is already crisscrossed with deep, angry fissures that throb and weep with lymph. Psoriatic stigmata. The scratching is carnal, shameful, animal. It is not merely scratching; it is ripping, digging, and tearing into skin, an attack of epidermal proportions and an attack on sanity itself.

The scratching is a response to the full-scale assault being waged by my overactive immune system. A system that releases a never-ending torrent of skin cells to the surface of my body every

 See jhupress.com/livingwithitch/ for a video interview with Krista K., who has psoriasis.

three or four days, quadruple the normal rate, where they pile up and pile up, layer after layer, sealing me in, stretching across my body parts like the hide on a native drum—tight, tense, and no longer animate.

When maximum tension is reached, when there can be no more buildup of cells, my skin splits open and terrible trenches are formed into which the seeds of itch are implanted. Beneath the surface, as the healing process begins, the seeds of itch sprout and bloom again and again in an endless crescendo of stimulus silently screaming for attention and the undeniable pleasure-pain of maniacal scratching. If I could peel away the entire top layer of skin to get to the origin of the itch, I would. So powerful is the urge.

But I can never find the origin. And since there is no origin, there is no end and there can be no real satisfaction. The cycle of psoriatic itch is endless and perfect in its process. A perfect mutation. A distorted signal from double helix to dermis, a menacing Morse code: crack, bleed, heal, itch, scratch, crack, bleed, heal, itch, scratch.

The whole affair is a frantic rave, a tiny, pulsing universe of collagenous and elastic fibers twisting and tangling, overwhelming my ability to resist the fall into frenzied scratching. When the frenzy finally stops, the devastation is complete. I have scratched myself to bleeding, and I will pay handsomely for it. The price is pain, and it is never in short supply. It is there before the itch and made worse after the scratching. It may wax and wane from time to time, from treatment to treatment, but it never really dissipates completely. When it does not strike like lightning, it is lurking around the corner, a mugger ready to assault a woman who has already been beaten. She is tired. She does not fight back.

Like any self-destructive behavior, in the beginning you can hide it. You want to hide it. You care about hiding it. You can find places to perform scratching sessions alone like a scaly, primordial beast. You can close your office door between meetings and scrape your palms over the edge of your desk like a lunatic. You can hide in the shower every day, weeping as you endure the barrage of stings, the spray invading every open crevice. When the stinging subsides and the skin begins to loosen, giving in just a little, you can employ pumice stones and files and fingernails to get at yourself, file yourself down, the evidence of the act safely circling the drain.

But the constant emotional weathering of chronic disease can wear a person down. The illusion of restraint is washed away like modesty in childbirth or many years of marriage. Soon enough, the scratching becomes a part of your persona, and you begin to believe that you are a person who cannot control herself, even in public. You become a person who will scratch her bloody feet in the living room, in front of family members, without even knowing she's doing it.

Adding to this humiliated state is the fallout of flakes, a wake of human dust that follows the psoriatic like the glittery trail of a Disney fairy, providing a constant stream of evidence of disease, both physical and psychological. There is flake fallout without the scratching, but the scratching only intensifies the plume, like a toddler shaking a snow globe over a tile floor, capricious and unheeding, creating a blizzard over a tiny alpine town.

To me, my itchy flakes are revolting. I carry them around on my hands all day long. I walk around with them in my shoes day in and day out. I scratch them out of my scalp. I am covered, perhaps not all over, but certainly in places where it counts. During particularly bad flares, there are other unspeakable places that also crack, bleed, and itch and must be scratched. This is the emotional coup de grace. The mortification is so complete, so personal, and so base that it is difficult to feel whole and human at times. It is easy to feel ugly. It is easy to feel like there is more at stake than your skin.

I am embarrassed by my skin. I am embarrassed by my incessant scratching. Relentless itch and constant pain are a part of my identity. Every time I hide my hands in shame, every time someone catches me picking and scratching at myself, every time I look at myself in the mirror, I try to convince myself that my psoriasis is only skin deep.

A Note to Readers about Coping

In recent years, the introduction of biologic medications and other treatments has made a significant difference in the lives of people living with the pain and itch of psoriasis. While no one treatment provides universal efficacy, there are many more options out there, including over-the-counter ointments and sprays made specifically to address itch. I have drawers full of them. Eucerin Itch Relief Spray is particularly helpful for me. In general, keeping my skin moisturized with good old Vaseline is a way of life. Anything to combat the dry, tight feeling. I am in a constant battle to prevent itchy cracks and then to soothe them when the battle has been lost. Applying ointments and medications to damp skin is most effective. Beyond the physical, getting educated about the disease and connecting with others who share my experience has made a world of difference, as well. Just knowing that I am not alone in the fight can provide relief. Volunteering with the National Psoriasis Foundation, finding the right partner in my dermatologist, and telling my story through writing and advocating for others are all ways that help me cope with the life-altering effects of chronic pain and itch.

4
Psoriasis

What Is Psoriasis?

Psoriasis is a common skin condition affecting 1 or 2% of the population. People with psoriasis have chronic red lesions that are often raised and thick, with an upper layer of flaky white scale (figure 4.1). Psoriasis can appear on any area of the body but frequently affects the elbows, knees, scalp, trunk, and genital region. While we will mainly focus on **plaque** psoriasis, since this is the most common form, other types of psoriasis include *erythrodermic* (severe redness spanning a large surface area), *guttate* (smaller red spots appearing together on the skin), *pustular* (white blisters surrounded by areas of redness), and *inverse* (skin redness occurs in body folds such as the groin and armpits).

Did you know?

"Psoriasis" comes from the Greek word "psora," meaning "itch." Indeed, itch is often a devastating symptom in people with psoriasis. For them, the itching is an inseparable part of the condition.

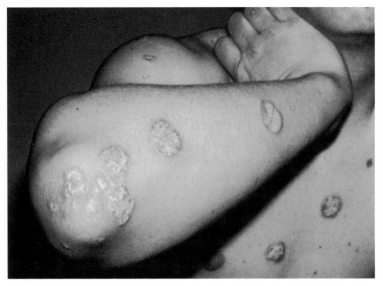

Figure 4.1. Classic lesion of psoriasis featuring scaly, flaky, white **plaques** on the elbows. © National Psoriasis Foundation.

Itch in Psoriasis

Itch is a very common symptom of psoriasis. In fact, itch affects the vast majority of people with psoriasis. People with psoriasis often suffer from generalized itch that can significantly affect their quality of life and sleep.

While itch in any skin condition can be vexing, itch in psoriasis is a cause for special concern because scratching to alleviate itch associated with psoriasis may increase the development of future skin lesions and cause flare-ups of psoriasis. Indeed, areas of the skin in psoriasis that are affected by trauma (such as by scratching) are more likely to develop new psoriatic skin lesions in the same region. The appearance of lesions in areas of trauma is known as the *Koebner phenomenon* or *Koebnerization*. Areas of the skin that are particularly itchy in people with psoriasis include the scalp, buttocks, umbilicus (belly button), and genital region.

Table 4.1 Treatments for psoriatic itch

Psoriatic itch	Medication
Treatments shown to improve psoriatic itch	Topical: capsaicin, topical salicylates Systemic: phototherapy, cyclosporine, biologicals (etanercept, infliximab, adalimumab, ustekinumab)
Suggested treatments for psoriatic itch	Topical: Pramoxine, topical salicylates plus topical steroids Systemic: Methotrexate, Mirtazapine, Paroxetine, Fluvoxamine, Gabapentin, Pregabalin, Butorphanol, Naltrexone, Aprepitant

Source: Adopted from Valdes-Rodriguez R, Kwatra SG, Yosipovitch G. "Itch in Psoriasis: From Basic Mechanisms to Practical Treatments" *Psoriasis Forum* 18, no. 3 (2012).

Treating Itch Associated with Psoriasis

The goal for itch treatment in people with psoriasis is to break the vicious "itch-scratch cycle." Many general treatments for psoriasis are also effective in relieving psoriatic itch. Some of the medications have a significant effect on improving people's itch even before their skin lesions improve. These agents include a new class of drugs called *biologicals,* a term describing agents that work by targeting specific parts of the body's immune system. A complete list of medications that may improve psoriatic itch is provided in table 4.1. (More detailed descriptions of many of these agents are provided in chapters 14 and 15, which describe treatments commonly used to alleviate itch.)

A Patient's Perspective
Cutaneous Lymphoma Itch

Itching was something I never gave a second thought to for much of my life. A few cases of poison ivy or bug bites were the extent of my experience with itch. That is until I developed a rash around my waist at the ripe old age of thirty-one and was diagnosed with a rare form of lymphoma called mycosis fungoides. This is a form of cutaneous lymphoma, treatable, but not curable, and becomes a chronic disease that needs to be managed over the course of one's lifetime. The initial itching wasn't too bad early on as it was confined to a mild rash, and with proper treatment (photochemotherapy), the annoyance of the itching subsided. It wasn't something that I thought much about again until my disease transformed, and I began to break out in lesions on many areas of my body.

This type of itch was beyond anything I had ever experienced before. It was intense and nonstop. Think for a moment of the inside of your skin feeling like it was on fire, with an itch so intense that the only way to make it go away is to scratch until your skin bleeds. It was the only way I could get relief. As my disease progressed, we tried different therapies, but none worked

 See jhupress.com/livingwithitch/ for a video interview with Susan T., who has cutaneous lymphoma.

at all on the intense itching. I didn't sleep for more than two years. Nights were the worst time. I tried all kinds of meditation, ways to calm myself, take my mind off of the incessant itching, but nothing worked until I scratched. In the middle of the night, I would scream out because I couldn't take the feeling of thousands of ants crawling all over my body. Cold compresses, oatmeal baths, ice cube baths, every topical known to man didn't work.

I remember playing a game with myself as I drove my car, how long can I count before I have to scratch some part of my body to relieve the itch. It takes over your life.

For me, the ultimate treatment of electron beam radiation eradicated my lesions and tumors but, more important, resolved the itch. I count myself as one of the lucky patients living with mycosis fungoides and without the itch now that my disease is under control. Unfortunately, there are many patients who have not found a solution to this intense itching. For those who live with this extreme sensation day by day, finding a solution to the itching is just as important as finding a cure for this currently incurable disease. Living with a chronic form of cancer is hard enough, but, when you add on top of that living with uncontrollable itching, it makes life so much harder. I excused myself many times from social events to spend time in the bathroom scratching and then trying to stop the bleeding so I could go back to the event, hoping no one would notice. Not only is this an intense physical experience, it is also an emotional one. Trying to hide the scratching when it is so intense takes a toll on your self-esteem as well as your ability to deal with the disease itself. You are always looking for a place to hide and scratch or a post to scratch your back on, like a bear. It's embarrassing to say the least. I spent so much of my time trying to find ways to scratch that were not noticeable. Or needing to use some kind of implement like a yard stick or kitchen tool to get to a hard to reach place.

It is mortifying when people notice that you are constantly itching. I remember one time when my boss commented about my excessive itching. I was horrified and became even more self-conscious. It takes a big toll on your life and enjoyment.

Trying to describe to other people how it feels to itch this way is very hard. Unless you have experienced it for yourself, you really can't imagine how it feels. It is also not a topic I wanted to talk to anyone about. Living with this kind of itching along with a rare disease is very lonely. Many times clinicians don't fully appreciate the impact the itching has on day-to-day life. It is not the "main" disease that is being treated, so often I found that there was not much discussion on how to manage this component of my disease. To say this is frustrating would not be doing justice to how I felt at the time. Sleepless, in pain, and feeling alone made for a very difficult time in my life. Fortunately for me, the intensity of the itching only lasted a few years. For many others living with cutaneous lymphoma, this is not the case. Finding help not only for the physical itching itself is important but also for the other emotional components that go along with this kind of day-to-day trauma.

Today I have the privilege of talking with other patients living with cutaneous lymphomas and dealing with itch. There are as many ways of dealing with the itch as there are people living with the itch. The only way to know what might work is to try everything that is available. I can only share my experience and what worked best for me. I encourage patients to connect through the Cutaneous Lymphoma Foundation and find other patients they can talk with. It helps to know that you are not alone in dealing with this. It is also important to get additional emotional help or support to deal with the non-physical side effects of living with cutaneous lymphoma and itch.

Hopefully, one day the research will show the underlying cause of the itch and ultimately provide a way to manage this debilitating disease side effect. In the meantime, I am grateful to be relatively itch-free today and only hope that this will continue so that I can live my life to the fullest. I wish for all patients that they too can find a resolution to this debilitating malady so they can live their lives fully.

5

Cutaneous T-cell Lymphoma

What Is Cutaneous T-cell Lymphoma?

Cutaneous T-cell lymphoma (CTCL) is a highly uncommon form of skin cancer that affects the immune system. The prevalence of CTCL in the United States is between 16,000 and 20,000 cases. The disease is more common in people older than fifty, and it affects nearly twice as many men as women. Cancer in CTCL originates from cells known as *T lymphocytes,* which are a type of white blood cell. These cells are members of the immune system and have several functions, including playing critical roles in identifying and attacking infections.

In people with CTCL, T lymphocytes have mutations that cause them to accumulate in the skin, which in turn causes different types of skin lesions. CTCL first appears as lesions in areas of the skin that are usually protected from sun exposure. In lighter-skinned people, these lesions are red and scaly patches. In people with darker skin color, lesions in the skin often appear as either very dark (*hyperpigmented*) or light (*hypopigmented*).

Different Forms of CTCL

There are several forms of CTCL. Of these, the two most common subtypes of CTCL are *mycosis fungoides* and *Sézary* syndrome.

Mycosis fungoides (figure 5.1) is the most common form of CTCL. People with mycosis fungoides often have localized areas of red, itchy patches in areas protected from the sun that are often confused with eczema or psoriasis.

Sézary syndrome is a variety of CTCL (considered to be a more advanced form of mycosis fungoides) that is characterized by the spread of mutated T cells into the bloodstream. People

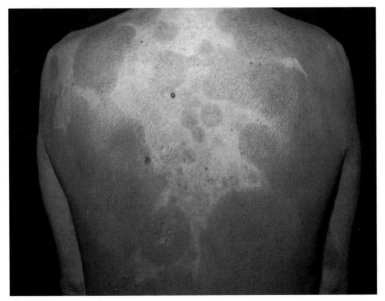

Figure 5.1. Patient with extensive mycosis fungoides, a form of skin cancer known as cutaneous T-cell lymphoma. Image appears with permission from VisualDx © Logical Images, Inc.

Table 5.1. Systemic treatments that may improve itch associated with cutaneous T-cell lymphoma (CTCL)

Therapy	Description
Phototherapy	Different forms include narrow-band ultraviolet B (UVB) and psoralen plus ultraviolet A (PUVA).
Denileukin difitox	This drug targets a **receptor** on cells that binds a specific cytokine (substances secreted by immune cells), known as interleukin-2.
Alemtuzumab	An antibody that targets lymphocytes that have a specific marker known as CD-52.
Histone deacetylase (HDAC) inhibitors	These drugs, which include Vorinostat and Romidepsin, work through modulating the expression of genes.
Gabapentin and mirtazapine	These drugs work primarily on the central nervous system and are further discussed in chapter 15.
Aprepitant	This drug is an FDA-approved agent used for chemotherapy-induced nausea and vomiting that can also be effective in CTCL-induced pruritus. It works by blocking a receptor on the cell membrane (known as neurokinin-1), which is now seen as possibly being linked to itch.
Methotrexate	This is a common anticancer medication (also very commonly used to treat psoriasis) that works by interfering with DNA synthesis.
Extracorporeal photopheresis	For this therapy, first a person's blood is drawn, then the blood is treated with specific chemicals and exposed to ultraviolet light, and subsequently the blood is returned back to the person.
Thalidomide	This anticancer agent inhibits the transmission of itch in nerves.

with Sézary syndrome usually have an extremely itchy, scaling red rash that covers most of their body.

Itch in CTCL

Itch is a particularly intractable feature of CTCL. Indeed, it is often the first and most bothersome symptom of CTCL and can significantly affect quality of life and sleep (see the patient's perspective on CTCL, which appears before this chapter). Studies have estimated that the incidence of itch in CTCL patients ranges between 66 and 88%. Itch is more common in people with Sézary syndrome than in those with mycosis fungoides. It is also significantly more common in later stages of the disease. The itch is usually generalized, but it can also be localized to specific skin lesions.

Itch in CTCL is thought to be caused by the release of substances secreted by cells in the immune system called **cytokines**. Cytokines are released by T lymphocytes and are present at increased levels in the skin of people who have CTCL. While there is no cure for itch associated with CTCL, several treatment options exist that may help.

Treating Itch Associated with CTCL

Itch in people with CTCL can be a chronic problem that is severe and may be unresponsive to treatment. First-line treatments for people with CTCL who suffer from severe itch include emollients (moisturizers), topical high-potency steroids, and oral antihistamines (these are discussed in more detail in chapters 14 and 15). In addition, wet dressings are also effective in treating itch associated with CTCL (also discussed in chapter 14). However, these antipruritic therapies are usually only effective in the earliest stages of disease, if at all. In general, the management of CTCL-related itch is based upon treating the lymphoma. Systemic therapies that have been shown to improve itch in people with CTCL are included in table 5.1.

6

Chronic Urticaria

What Is Chronic Urticaria?

Urticaria is another word for hives, which are red, very itchy, raised bumps of the skin. These elevated lesions can come and go over a period of only a few hours. Chronic urticaria is the term used to describe the presence of hives for longer than six weeks; the hives may go away, but they frequently come back. Chronic urticaria affects women more than men; as much as 3% of the population may be affected at some point in their lives.

One subgroup of chronic urticaria are the physical urticarias, in which hives are caused by a pressure on the skin. Among the physical urticarias, the most common form is *dermatographism,* literally "skin writing," in which the skin can become raised and inflamed and itchy when rubbed or scratched (figure 6.1).

Another subgroup is called *cholinergic urticaria,* which refers to smaller hive-like lesions that are surrounded by areas of inflamed skin; cholinergic urticaria often occurs as a result of body heat and sweating, whether due to exercise, stress, heat from the sun, certain spicy foods, and many other causes.

Another important subgroup of chronic urticaria is *chron-*

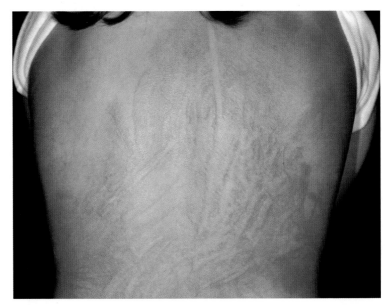

Figure 6.1. Chronic urticaria (hives) with dermatographism, also referred as "skin writing." Dermatographism appears as localized swelling with itch in areas that are rubbed or stroked. Image appears with permission from VisualDx © Logical Images, Inc.

ic spontaneous urticaria, when the urticaria is not linked to any apparent specific physical stimulus. In most cases the cause is unknown, though it can be associated with autoimmune conditions (diseases where the body attacks itself).

Itch Associated with Chronic Urticaria

Itch is a common feature in people affected by chronic urticaria. In these people, histamine is an important cause of itch. Indeed, in urticaria there are specific cells known as **mast cells** (see chapter 1) that are present on the surface of the skin and that often release their contents (a concept referred to as *degranulation*), which includes histamine and other inflammatory substances. The release of histamine, which binds to histamine **receptors**, subsequently causes inflammation in the surrounding skin areas.

Table 6.1. Systemic treatments that may improve itch associated with chronic urticaria

Treatment	Description
Histamine receptor antagonists (blockers)	These medications work through blocking the release of histamine by acting on the histamine **receptor** in the cell membrane. Several subtypes are discussed below.
H1 receptor antagonists	These medications work through blocking a specific subtype of the histamine receptor known as H1.
First-generation antihistamines (examples: hydroxyzine, diphenhydramine)	These medications are a class of H1 receptor antagonists that cross the blood-brain barrier and are often very sedating.
Second-generation antihistamines (examples: cetirizine, loratadine)	These medications are H1 receptor antagonists that tend to be longer acting, have a slower onset of action, and in general are less sedating than first-generation antihistamines.
Third-generation antihistamines (examples: Fexofenadine, Levocetirizine, Desloratadine)	These medications are H1 antagonists very similar to second-generation antihistamines but with slightly increased efficacy and fewer adverse drug reactions.
Leukotriene antagonists (examples: montelukast, zileuton)	These medications are used frequently by allergists to treat urticaria, but their efficacy is questionable. They work by blocking the action of substances known as leukotrienes, compounds produced by the immune system that contribute to inflammation.

continued

Treating Itch Associated with Chronic Urticaria

Most forms of chronic urticaria do not have a specific cause, but urticaria can be aggravated by certain triggers, including stress, sunlight exposure, and certain types of weather, clothing, and foods that liberate histamine, such as seafood. Keeping a journal and documenting the circumstances surrounding episodes might be helpful in finding out what factors are specifically related to urticaria. In terms of pharmacological treatment, since urticaria-induced itch is related to the release of histamine, the first-line treatment for chronic urticaria is the use of both

Treatment	Description
Oral corticosteroids	These medications reduce the activity of the immune system and are not directly treating itch. However, since they reduce inflammation, they also can decrease itch. These medications are intended only for short-term use during periods of disease exacerbation (see chapter 15).
Cyclosporine	Cyclosporine is an oral medication that suppresses an overactive immune system. This medication works on T lymphocytes to reduce the amount of **cytokine** secreted by cells (see chapter 15).
Mycophenolate mofetil	Mycophenolate mofetil is a drug that suppresses the immune system. The most common side effects are gastrointestinal symptoms including diarrhea and nausea.
Hydroxychloroquine	This is an anti-inflammatory medication that works on the immune system and has been shown to be effective in some forms of chronic urticaria. It may be effective in reducing itch though suppressing the immune system.
Dapsone/sulfasalazine/ colchicine	These medications mostly work on neutrophil activation.
Methotrexate	Oral anticancer drug that can be used to suppress the immune system. This medication inhibits DNA synthesis.
IV Immunoglobulin	These medications are antibodies (molecules that bind to other small compounds) that inhibit immunoglobulins (substances that activate the inflammatory response).

first-generation and second-generation antihistamines (these are briefly discussed in table 6.1 and in chapter 15, on treatments). Many people respond to antihistamines, but there is still a significant portion of patients who do not respond to antihistamine therapy. Table 6.1 discusses all the current systemic treatments that may be effective in alleviating itch associated with chronic urticaria.

7
Neuropathic Itch

Neuropathic itch, or nerve itch, includes a broad group of conditions in which itch is caused by damage to nerve fibers that occurs at different levels. Any localized itch with limited body involvement and without rash should raise the suspicion of neuropathic itch.

Neuropathy, or damage to nerve fibers, can be classified into two categories: *peripheral* and *central*. Peripheral nerve fiber damage can be defined as damage to nerves occurring at any point beyond the spinal cord where the nerves branch out. Central nerve fiber damage includes any damage to nerves in the spinal cord or brain.

Peripheral Neuropathic Itch
Postherpetic neuralgia

Postherpetic neuralgia classically features pain in certain parts of the body as a result of nerve damage caused by the varicella zoster virus. This virus causes chicken pox in children and can lie dormant in a person's nervous system for many years. In approximately 10 to 20% of adults, the varicella zoster virus reactivates and causes severe burning pain. Many also experience neuropathic itch. Itch is more common in the face, neck, and head. The best treatments for itch associated with postherpetic neuralgia are medications specifically targeting the nerves, such as gabapentin and pregabalin.

Brachioradial pruritus

Brachioradial pruritus is a localized itch of the upper arms, forearms, and elbows that can start in one or both arms and is often of a burning and stinging nature. It seems to originate as a spinal nerve pathology affecting the cervical (neck) nerve roots (those thought to be responsible for symptoms are located between the C4 and C7 cervical vertebrae). Brachioradial pruritus has specifically been associated with impingement or traction of spinal nerves. It can become worse by exposure to sunlight. This kind of itch can also become widespread or spread to the rest of the body. Topical treatments that may be especially effective for patients with brachioradial pruritus include local anesthetics (such as lidocaine, prilocaine, or pramoxine) and topical capsaicin.

Notalgia paresthetica

Notalgia paresthetica is a form of chronic itch that is localized around the scapular area on the back. People with notalgia paresthetica have an intense urge to scratch the area underneath the shoulder blade. In addition to itch, people can experience tingling and burning sensations, and the area is sometimes hyperpigmented (dark) as a consequence of scratching for so many years. Similar to brachioradial pruritus, notalgia paresthetica originates with anything that may affect the spinal nerves (ranging from degenerative changes to nerve impingement). Here the thoracic

Did you know?

Sometimes patients with brachioradial pruritus, notalgia paresthetica, and other forms of neuropathic (nerve) itch can get relief from the application of an ice pack to the areas of affected skin. The ice pack is thought to work by chilling the skin to the point of numbness. This dramatic temperature change may alleviate itch by activating cold nerve fibers. This treatment has been called the "ice-pack sign."

nerves are affected (the specific nerves affected are thought to be located between the thoracic vertebrae numbered T2 and T6). Topical treatments usually provide some relief in people with notalgia paresthetica and include capsaicin and local anesthetics. Physical therapy may also provide some relief.

Central Neuropathic Itch

Central neuropathic itch involves pathology in the brain or spinal cord. Descriptions of two examples of central causes of itch follow.

Multiple sclerosis

Multiple sclerosis is a disease in which the fatty sheath around nerve fibers in the spinal cord and brain is damaged. People with multiple sclerosis have reported outbreaks of itch that can spontaneously occur (sometimes for seconds to minutes) and can be of an extreme intensity.

Stroke

Numerous brain areas have been found to be associated with itch, thus infarction of brain tissue as a result of a stroke can lead to significant itch.

8

Itch Associated with Autoimmune Disorders

Bullous Skin Disorders
What are bullous skin disorders?

Bullous skin disorders refer to the development of blisters, which are collections of fluid between different layers in the skin. The majority of these diseases are types of autoimmune disorders, in which the immune system attacks the body. An example of these disorders is gluten intolerance, which can produce dermatitis herpetiformis (figure 8.1). What distinguishes each of these disorders from the others is the level in the skin where the blister forms. On the one hand, the deeper the layer of the skin where the blister forms, the more tense the blister will be (one example is bullous pemphigoid; figure 8.2). On the other hand, the more superficial the area of the skin where the blister forms, the more likely it is for the lesion to be flaccid or easily peel off (for example, pemphigus; figure 8.3). Thus, the different diseases can be grouped based on the level of the skin where blisters form, along with their distribution in the body.

Itch in bullous skin disorders

The bullous disorders that are most commonly associated with itch include the following:

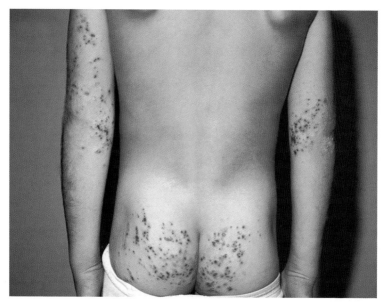

Figure 8.1. Classic lesions of dermatitis herpetiformis, featuring redness of the skin and an eruption composed of tiny blisters known as vesicles on the arms, elbows, and buttocks. These lesions can cause severe itching. Image appears with permission from VisualDx © Logical Images, Inc.

▶ *Bullous pemphigoid (BP).* Blisters in bullous pemphigoid are tense and difficult to break. Bullous pemphigoid often begins with terrible itch that can be generalized or limited to several parts of the body. Itch can precede lesions in BP and is often the most troubling symptom for people who have BP.

▶ *Dermatitis herpetiformis.* Dermatitis herpetiformis is often associated with gluten intolerance. It is symmetrical and often consists of blisters, **erosions**, and **papules** found commonly on the buttocks, elbows, and knees. Dermatitis herpetiformis is characterized by an extremely severe form of itching. Usually it's not blisters that you see, but rather small erosions and **excoriations** that can be confused with eczema or other secondary skin changes. Itch in dermatitis herpetiformis can also appear before the skin lesions.

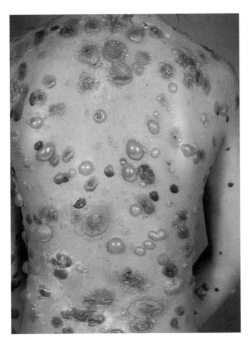

Figure 8.2. A case of bullous pemphigoid, a rare skin condition that causes large, fluid-filled blisters. Image appears with permission from VisualDx © Logical Images, Inc.

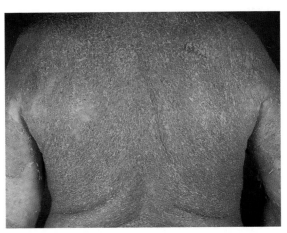

Figure 8.3. Extensive **erosions** on the back from pemphigus foliaceus, one of the itchiest autoimmune blistering disorders. Image appears with permission from VisualDx © Logical Images, Inc.

▶ *Pemphigus foliaceus.* One of the itchiest autoimmune blistering disorders, pemphigus foliaceus often affects the face and chest and back (the blisters are usually not found in the mucus membranes). Pemphigus foliaceus has blisters that often rupture and leave behind **erosions**.

▶ *Epidermolysis bullosa congenita.* This is a rare inherited disease (incidence is 1 in 50,000 individuals) that causes the formation of blisters in the skin and mucous membranes. The skin in people with epidermolysis bullosa is extremely fragile, and even minimal trauma or friction can cause significant blistering. There are many genetic variants of epidermolysis bullosa. One is epidermolysis bullosa pruriginosa, which is a rare dystrophic variant that produces uncontrollable itching and scratching, often leading to disfiguring skin lesions. Read more about epidermolysis bullosa and its various forms at http://www.debra.org.

Specific treatments for itch associated with bullous disorders

Many general antipruritic therapies are also effective in reducing itch in people with bullous diseases (see chapters 14 and 15). Most medications that treat specific diseases that result in bullous disorders also are effective in reducing itch. For example, oral corticosteroids can be very effective at relieving itch by suppressing the inflammatory response. Dapsone is an antibacterial agent useful in reducing inflammation and in reducing itch in people who have dermatitis herpetiformis. Its anti-inflammatory (and likely antipruritic effect) comes from its blocking of *myeloperoxidase*, a protein that is expressed in neutrophils, which is a type of inflammatory cell predominant in skin lesions in people who have dermatitis herpetiformis. Dapsone may also be effective in treating people with bullous pemphigoid.

Dermatomyositis
What is dermatomyositis?

Dermatomyositis is an inflammatory disease characterized by symmetrical muscle weakness and significant skin rash. The rash

Did you know?

Gottron's sign is one of the most common skin manifestations of *dermatomyositis*, Gottron's sign manifests as a red, scaly eruption over the knuckles, elbows, or knee joints. Image appears with permission from VisualDx © Logical Images, Inc.

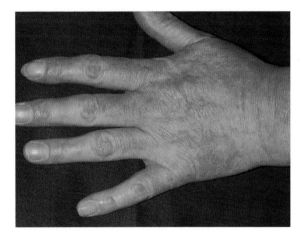

in dermatomyositis is aggravated by sun exposure and features a violaceous, or purplish, rash usually on the eyelids, face, neck, knuckles, or elbows.

Dermatomyositis can be associated with an underlying malignancy in some people. Muscle weakness often first affects the hips and shoulders and can cause difficulty in climbing stairs or standing from a sitting position.

Itch in dermatomyositis

Itch is one of the most bothersome symptoms encountered by people with dermatomyositis. A recent study among people with dermatomyositis conducted both in the United States and Singapore found itch to be the most common initial symptom in both populations.

Treatment for itch associated with dermatomyositis

Dermatomyositis is associated with high levels of inflammation (which is a factor in increased itch). Thus, general treatments that reduce inflammation, such as oral or topical corticosteroids, may be an effective treatment for reducing itch along with improving muscle function. Other agents that suppress the immune system, such as Tacrolimus, also are effective in reducing itch through a similar mechanism.

Other Autoimmune Disorders

Other autoimmune disorders often featuring itch include scleroderma, Sjogren's syndrome, and hyperthyroidism (among numerous others).

9

Itch Associated with Infections

Many infections have the potential to cause severe itch. In this chapter, we discuss a select group of infections that feature a particularly strong association with itch.

Scabies

What is scabies?

Scabies is an extremely itchy condition that affects as many as 300 million people worldwide. It is characterized by skin infestation of the mite *Sarcoptes scabiei*. This mite is tiny, often burrowing and laying its eggs in the skin. Scabies is acquired through direct body-to-body contact with another individual (usually this contact is prolonged). For this reason it is more common in children attending day-care centers, in nursing home residents, and in family members of people who are affected with the condition.

While the face is spared from scabies, most other areas of the body are not so fortunate. Scabies most commonly affects the skin folds including the neck, armpits, genitals, and finger web areas (figure 9.1).

Scabies can often be difficult for doctors to diagnose, since it often mimics many other skin diseases. If several family members also suffer from severe itch, then a diagnosis of scabies

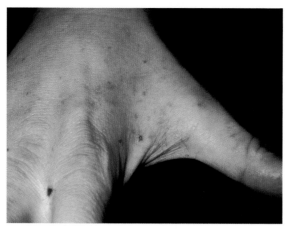

Figure 9.1. Scabies on hands in the folds between the fingers, a common sign that mites can be found. Image appears with permission from VisualDx © Logical Images, Inc.

should be made until proven otherwise (even if the rash does not look classical).

When scabies is suspected, doctors often scrape the skin folds of the hands and look under the microscope to see if any mites are present.

Itch in scabies

Severe itching is the hallmark of scabies. Itch in scabies tends to be worse in the evening and at night. The itch of scabies is caused by an allergic reaction to mite proteins and can continue for several weeks to months after the mites have been eliminated (called *post-scabetic itch*). Since the itch in scabies is secondary to an allergic reaction, if scabies is contracted again, the intense itch will immediately return due to an immune response.

 Did you know?
The name scabies originates from the Latin word "scabere" for "scratch."

Treatment for itch associated with scabies

Treatment is with medications known as scabicides, which aim to eradicate the mite. These include permethrin cream, oral ivermectin, or crotamiton (known to have a significant effect in reducing itch). In addition, other general antipruritic treatments including sedating antihistamines can also be beneficial.

Dermatophytosis

Dermatophytes (superficial fungal infections, also known as *tinea infections*, or ringworm) are common causes of itch that is localized to specific body areas. These infections often start as red scaly patches that have central clearing. These infections are especially common in athletes and tend to affect the skin folds, such as in the groin area ("jock itch") and the feet ("athlete's foot"). Predisposing factors include clothing that is tight-fitting, warm temperature, and moisture. Itch associated with tinea infections can be severe and cause significant distress.

Treatment—usually antifungal medications—for itch associated with fungal infections is directed against the underlying cause. Common topical antifungals include miconazole, terbinafine, clotrimazole, and ketoconazole. In more severe cases (or in infections affecting the scalp or nails), systemic treatment with oral antifungal medications is used.

Folliculitis

Folliculitis (as the name implies) is the infection of one or more hair follicles and can occur anywhere on the skin that hair is present (thus it does not occur on the palms of the hands or soles of the feet). Folliculitis happens when hair follicles (which

Did you know?

Another name for dermatophytosis is ringworm, but this is a misnomer! The infection isn't caused by worms at all but rather is the result of a fungal infection.

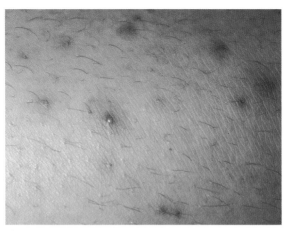

Figure 9.2. Folliculitis, or inflammation of the hair follicle, on trunk. Image appears with permission from VisualDx © Logical Images, Inc.

are often damaged through touching, rubbing, or shaving) become infected with *Staph* bacteria (short for *Staphylococcus*). Pimples or pustules (which are full of pus) are the result of these infected follicles (figure 9.2). Itch in folliculitis can be significant and is partly due to inflammation that occurs because of the infection. In addition, *Staphylococcus bacteria* can activate **proteases** that also induce itch (see chapter 3).

Warm compresses may help drain the infected follicles but the best treatment for folliculitis is antibacterial therapy. Common topical antibiotics used to treat folliculitis include clindamycin and mupirocin.

Human Immunodeficiency Virus

Itch is a common complaint of people with human immunodeficiency virus (HIV) (affecting between 30 and 60% of patients)

Did you know?

Folliculitis—an infection of hair follicles—that is caused by the bacterium *Staphylococcus aureus* is known as a "hot tub rash" and associated with sitting in dirty hot tubs.

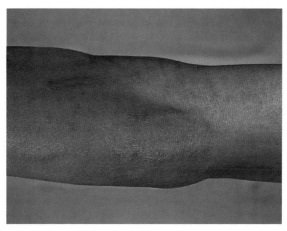

Figure 9.3. Dry skin itch in HIV patient. Image appears with permission from VisualDx © Logical Images, Inc.

and can be associated with HIV at many points of infection. Most commonly itch is an initial symptom or it presents as a consequence of dry skin (figure 9.3), which is a significant problem in people with HIV.

Primary skin disorders that are particularly common in HIV patients include psoriasis and seborrheic dermatitis (dandruff). Often, people present with itchy bumps of unknown origin—these can range from hypersensitivity reactions to insect bites to a disease that is particularly associated with advanced HIV known as *eosinophilic folliculitis*. This condition is characterized by small bumps that often affect many areas of the skin, including the trunk, back, face, and extremities. Treatment for itch associated with HIV infection is directed toward the underlying cause with highly active antiretroviral therapy (HAART), which usually combines at least three medications.

Onchocerciasis

Onchocerciasis is an infectious disease caused by the parasite *Onchocerca volvulus* (a roundworm). The majority of these infections occur in sub-Saharan Africa (in fact there are no reported cases in the Western Hemisphere). Around 18 million people suffer from this disease in Africa. This disease is known to cause intense, severe itching, although its most well-known aftereffect is blindness. Oral Ivermectin is the treatment of choice and is able to kill the parasite.

10

Itch Associated with Systemic Disorders

Itch can be caused by several systemic diseases of the human body that are not associated with a primary skin rash. People with systemic causes of itch often have secondary signs of scratching including the following: excoriations, lichenification, and prurigo nodules.

▶ *Excoriations* are abrasions on the surface of the skin due to chronic scratching (figure 10.1)

▶ *Lichenification* is thickening and hardening of the skin often due to chronic scratching and rubbing (these areas often have exaggerated skin markings; figure 10.2)

▶ *Prurigo nodules* are itchy bumps on the skin surface that are caused by chronic scratching (figure 10.3)

Uremic Pruritus
What is uremic pruritus?

Uremic pruritus is itch that is caused by chronic kidney disease (also known as end-stage renal failure, or ESRF) in people who are close to requiring dialysis or are currently undergoing dialysis. Uremic pruritus is usually generalized but can be especially severe on the back and the extremities. It can significantly

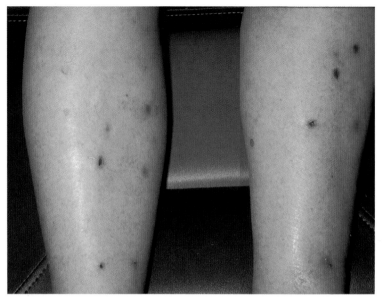

Figure 10.1. Excoriations, or an injury to a surface of the body caused by scratching. Image appears with permission from VisualDx © Logical Images, Inc.

affect quality of life, as it commonly produces sleep and mood disturbances.

People with uremic pruritus often have secondary signs of scratching such as heavily excoriated skin, lichenification, and prurigo nodules (described above).

What causes uremic pruritus?

The cause of uremic pruritus is still poorly understand, but it has been linked to imbalances in the immune and opioid systems, damage to nerve fibers transmitting itch, the release of **cytokines** during hemodialysis, and an abnormality in a number of laboratory values such as calcium and phosphorus that may be altered in people with chronic renal disease who are undergoing hemodialysis. (For more on laboratory tests, see pages 96–97.)

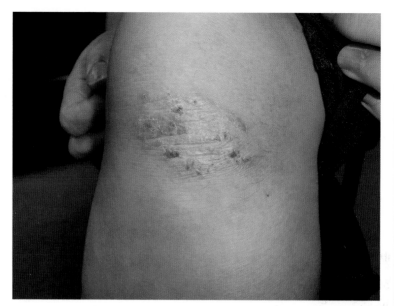

Figure 10.2. Lichenification, or thickening of the skin, with exaggeration of its normal markings. Courtesy of Dr. Hong Liang Tey.

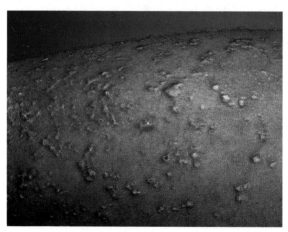

Figure 10.3. Prurigo nodules, an eruption of hard nodules in the skin, associated with intense itch. Image appears with permission from VisualDx © Logical Images, Inc.

Treating itch associated with uremic pruritus

Treatments for itch associated with uremic pruritus are limited, but several may provide some benefit. These include ultraviolet B (UVB) light and thalidomide (discussed in chapter 14). Other therapies that are effective include those that modulate the **opioid system**. Specifically, nalfurafine, currently approved in Japan for the treatment of uremic pruritus, has been shown to decrease both the intensity of itch as well as excoriations in hemodialysis patients. Since nerve fiber damage may also be involved, gabapentin and pregabalin have also been shown to be effective in the treatment of uremic pruritus.

In addition, people with uremic pruritus usually have especially dry skin that can be treated with moisturizers.

Pruritus of Cholestasis

What is pruritus of cholestasis?

Pruritus of cholestasis refers to itch associated with chronic liver disease. This itch is unique in that it often starts in the palms and soles and spreads to other body sites. Specific liver diseases associated with itch include hepatitis C, primary biliary cirrhosis (more common in women), intrahepatic cholestasis of pregnancy, and obstruction of the bile duct as a complication of cancers of the pancreas or biliary system.

What causes pruritus of cholestasis?

The exact cause of pruritus of cholestasis is currently unknown. However, studies have suggested a role for elevated levels of bile salts and opioid levels.

Treating itch associated with pruritus of cholestasis

Two therapies specific for pruritus of cholestasis include compounds that bind bile acids to lower their levels (examples are cholestyramine and ursodeoxycholic acid). Combining these treatments may be particularly helpful.

Pruritus Associated with Diseases of the Endocrine System

Disturbances in the endocrine system have the potential to cause significant itch and distress. Endocrine conditions that have been associated with pruritus are listed below. The best treatment for itch associated with these conditions is better disease control of the underlying condition.

Two conditions that can be associated with itch are thyroid problems and diabetes. While the exact mechanism is unknown, hyperthyroidism is more commonly associated with itch than hypothyroidism. Diabetes is a disease that results from increased levels of blood sugars. It has many potential complications, such as infections and damage to nerve fibers (neuropathy). One common infection in uncontrolled diabetes that is known to cause itch is candidal infection in skin folds. A candidal infection appears as a rapidly expanding red rash. Areas that are especially affected in people with diabetes include the skin folds and ano-genital region.

Neuropathy is a common complication in people with diabetes that can cause significant itch. One presentation for itch associated with diabetic neuropathy is lichen simplex chronicus, a localized itch that tends to affect the scalp and lower extremities. Lichen simplex chronicus may respond to treatment with topical capsaicin. In addition, a recent study from Japan showed that people with diabetic neuropathy have an increased frequency of itch affecting the trunk.

Pruritus Associated with Blood Disorders

Itch is a very common symptom in people with blood disorders. One form of blood disorder, cutaneous T-cell lymphoma, was discussed in chapter 5. Other lymphomas associated with itch include Hodgkin's and non-Hodgkin's lymphoma. Itch has also been associated with leukemias and other forms of erratic red and white blood cell production known as *myelodysplasia*.

Polycythemia vera is another blood disorder that is highly associated with itch, occurring in approximately half of all people with the condition. Itch in polycythemia vera is unique in that it is made worse and is often triggered by exposure to water. The cause of itch in polycythemia vera is unknown; it has been associated with increased levels of histamine.

11

Unique Types of Itch

Localized Itch

Many forms of itch (many of which have been discussed in previous chapters) are specific to certain body areas (see figure 11.1). Here we will detail types of itch affecting different parts of the body (progressing from top to bottom).

Scalp itch

The scalp is a very itchy area of the body. It is associated with inflammatory skin diseases such as seborrheic dermatitis (dandruff), psoriasis, and hair disorders such as the scarring alopecias (hair loss disorders) and lichen planus (see below). Finally, significant itch in the scalp can also occur as a consequence of nerve fiber damage (postherpetic neuralgia; see chapter 7).

Arm itch

As discussed in chapter 7, brachioradial pruritus is a form of localized itch that affects the arms. Liver disease also often first appears as itch in the palms before generalizing to other parts of the body.

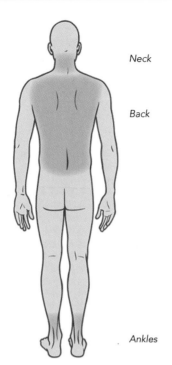

Figure 11.1. Areas prone to localized itch.

Neck

Back

Ankles

Genital itch

A common cause of genital itch in both sexes is allergic and irritant contact dermatitis (to underwear, for example), which is associated with a strong itching and burning sensation. Frictional dermatitis can also cause itch through excessive friction between skin surfaces (more commonly seen in obese individuals).

In addition, common dermatologic conditions including both atopic dermatitis and psoriasis can specifically affect the groin and genital regions. Finally, infectious diseases can also cause significant itch and include the following: candidiasis, herpes, scabies, and chlamydia.

Lichen simplex chronicus is another cause of genital itch in both men and women, which can be due to nerve fiber damage in the sacral region of the spinal cord and causes chronic scratch-

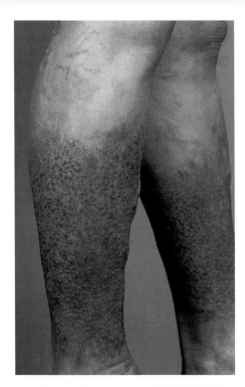

Figure 11.2. Lichen amyloidosis, itchy brownish **papules** commonly noted in lower legs. Courtesy of Dr. Hong Liang Tey.

ing and rubbing of the skin (resulting in thickening of the skin surface in this area). It is important to also mention here that the genital area is extremely sensitive due to abundant nerve fibers in the region. For this reason, specific treatments for genital itch include anesthetic lotions, which provide a numbing effect.

Leg itch

Itch (along with pain and burning sensations) in the legs has been associated with *chronic venous insufficiency*, a very common medical condition in the population that involves the pooling of blood in the legs.

Another common cause of itch in the legs in Asians and Hispanics is *lichen amyloidosis*, a condition characterized by small round lesions on the legs due to deposits of a protein called amyloid in the skin (figure 11.2).

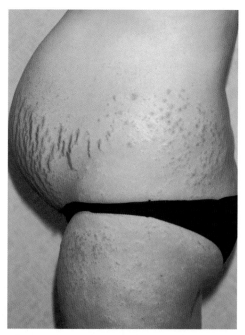

Figure 11.3. Polymorphic eruption of pregnancy is an itchy rash that develops during the third trimester of pregnancy that commonly begins on the abdomen, particularly within stretch marks. Image appears with permission from VisualDx © Logical Images, Inc.

Itch in Pregnancy

The types of skin conditions that can occur in pregnancy are detailed in table 11.1 and an example is shown in figure 11.3.

Itch and Menopause

Menopause is associated with a decrease in the amount of estrogen in the body and with changes in vaginal pH. Since estrogen receptors are also present on the skin, menopause is associated with significant changes in skin moisture and changes in its acidity (pH).

Atrophic vulvovaginitis is an itchy condition that can occur in menopausal and postmenopausal women and is associated with

Table 11.1. Causes of itch in pregnancy

Condition	Description
Polymorphic eruption of pregnancy	This condition, also known as pruritic urticarial papules and plaques of pregnancy, is characterized by very itchy welts and hives of the skin that typically begin in stretch marks located on the abdomen. It is associated with multiple pregnancies and weight gain. This rash typically occurs in late pregnancy or postpartum and usually resolves by 6 weeks after delivery (see figure 11.2).
Pemphigoid gestations	This is a rare autoimmune disease that involves the formation of very itchy red blisters and hives. In many cases the itch may begin before the appearance of skin lesions. This condition usually occurs in the third trimester or immediately postpartum and has a tendency to flare at the time of delivery. The condition typically resolves within weeks of delivery.
Intrahepatic cholestasis of pregnancy	This condition, frequently occurring in late pregnancy, is not associated with primary skin lesions. Instead, it is the result of an inability to effectively secrete bile salts (and is often diagnosed by an elevation of bile acids in the blood). Itch often occurs suddenly and starts on the palms of the hands or soles of the feet before quickly generalizing to the rest of the body. A specific treatment is ursodeoxycholic acid, which reduces serum bile acid levels.
Atopic eruption of pregnancy	This condition is associated with eczematous changes in the skin (preexisting atopic dermatitis is not a requirement). Unlike the other conditions mentioned above, atopic eruptions in pregnancy tend to occur earlier in the course of a pregnancy. Lesions take many forms and are often extremely itchy. Women with this condition often respond well to topical corticosteroids.

thinning of the vagina due to a decrease in estrogen levels. Many women with this condition quickly respond to topical therapy with estrogen.

Lichen sclerosus is another condition occurring after menopause that can affect the mucus membranes as well as the skin. It may appear as white and thinning of skin and white scarlike lesions

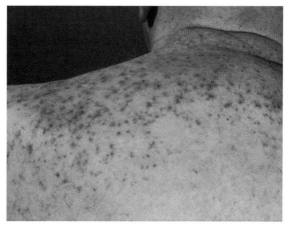

Figure 11.4. Grover's disease is a condition in which itchy red spots appear without warning, usually on a person's back or upper chest. Image appears with permission from VisualDx © Logical Images, Inc.

around the openings of the vagina and anus. Lichen sclerosus can be very itchy and is treated with topical corticosteroids (often the more potent types).

Itch in Older Adults

Advanced age often leads to an exacerbation of pruritic skin diseases. Older people are also more susceptible to a form of itch that is not attributed to a primary skin disorder. This is the disorder known as senile (or old age) pruritus, which can affect people older than sixty years but is more common in people in their seventies and eighties. The high prevalence of itch in this group can be attributed to physiological changes occurring in the skin as we age. These changes include a decrease in skin thickness and moisture, a gradual worsening of immune system function (known as *immunosenescence,* which can result in greater amounts of inflammation), and the frequent co-presence of psychological and neurodegenerative disorders. Specifically, age-related changes in nerve fibers and feelings of social isolation may exacerbate itch in this population.

Scabies (as mentioned previously) is also common because many older adults reside in long-term care facilities. This form of itch is often sudden in onset and severe in intensity.

Grover's disease (also known as *benign papular acantholytic dermatosis*) is another disease common in older people. Grover's disease occurs on the chest and back and is characterized by itchy red spots (figure 11.4).

It occurs more often in men, Caucasians, and those older than age fifty. Triggering factors for Grover's disease includes sweating, sunlight, and certain medications. Treatment is directed at making sure the skin is cool. Topical steroids can also be effective at treating lesions.

Swimmer's Itch

Swimmer's itch, also known as lake itch, often appears as itchy, red bumps on the lower extremities (figure 11.5). These skin lesions are the result of an immune reaction by the body against a waterborne parasite known as *schistosomatidae*. The larvae of these parasites enter the skin. Once in the skin these larvae immediately die and cause a reaction by the immune system that is often associated with significant inflammation. Each red bump corresponds to an area where a single parasite has invaded the skin.

Seabather's Eruption

Seabather's eruption is an extremely itchy rash that occurs underneath the bathing suits of people who swim and dive in the

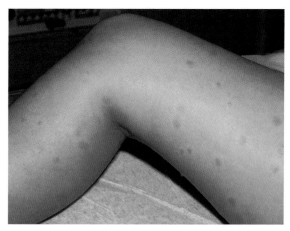

Figure 11.5. Swimmer's itch on lower extremities. It is an itchy skin rash caused by an allergic reaction to certain parasites. These microscopic parasites are released from infected snails into fresh water (such as lakes or ponds). Image appears with permission from VisualDx © Logical Images, Inc.

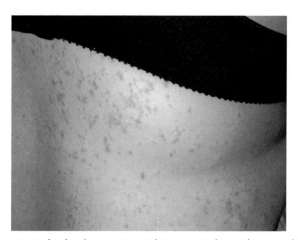

Figure 11.6. Seabather's eruption. This is an itchy rash caused by a hypersensitive reaction to the larval stage of a jellyfish. Image appears with permission from VisualDx © Logical Images, Inc.

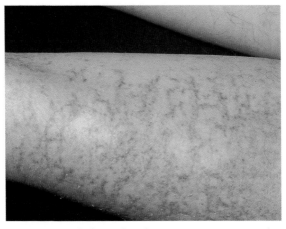

Figure 11.7. Winter itch from dry skin. Image appears with permission from VisualDx © Logical Images, Inc.

sea in tropical areas (figure 11.6). It is caused by a hypersensitivity reaction to the larval form of jellyfish.

Winter Itch

Winter itch describes a form of eczema in adults that is characterized by the skin becoming abnormally dry, itchy, and cracked during the winter months (figure 11.7). The lower legs and forearms tend to be especially affected. The treatment for winter itch is to regularly apply moisturizers and topical corticosteroid ointments.

Acne

Acne is a common condition that can affect people throughout the life span but is most common during adolescence (figure 11.8). Itch is a frequent component of acne. Indeed, a large Norwegian population study showed a significant correlation between the severity of acne and the intensity of itch. An explanation for this association is that severe acne is often inflammatory. In addition, the organism that causes acne is *Propionibacterium acnes*, which also produces many **proteases** that can activate the PAR-2 **receptor** (a known cause of itch, discussed in chapters 2 and 3).

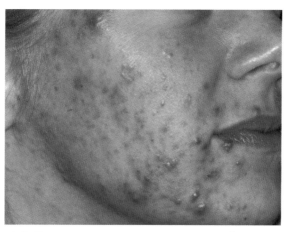

Figure 11.8. Inflammatory acne. Image appears with permission from VisualDx © Logical Images, Inc.

Itch and Burns or Scars

Scars from burns are highly associated with itch. Estimates of prevalence rates of itch three months after a burn injury are as high as 80 to 90%.

Itch and Keloids

Keloids are a type of scar that results in an overgrowth of scar tissue at the site of a healed skin injury (figure 11.9). Keloids often expand beyond the borders of a typical scar into normal skin and can be associated with a significant amount of itch, which is most common at the peripheral border of lesions.

Did you know?

Tetracycline, a common oral antibiotic used to treat acne, has the added benefit of reducing activation of the PAR-2 receptor, which is a chemical that acts to induce a biological response such as itch.

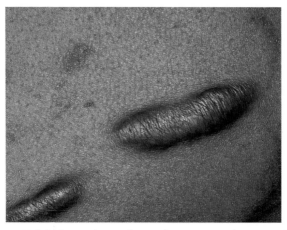

Figure 11.9. Keloid is an elevated scar that commonly causes itch. Image appears with permission from VisualDx © Logical Images, Inc.

Itch and Skin Cancer

Itch is a common feature accompanying nonmelanoma skin cancer, which includes both **basal cell** and **squamous cell carcinoma**. Less frequently, itch can also be associated with inflammatory types of melanoma.

Additional Inflammatory Skin Conditions: Lichen Planus

What is lichen planus?

Lichen planus (figure 11.10) is a common inflammatory disease that often results in an itchy rash of the skin or tender lesions in the mouth. In the skin, lesions of lichen planus are typically pink or purple in color and are most commonly located on the wrists and ankles. Lesions of lichen planus, both in the skin and in the mouth, often have a lace-like pattern on the surface composed of whitish lines known as Wickham striae. The cause of lichen planus is often unknown, but it has been linked to hepatitis C infection in some patients.

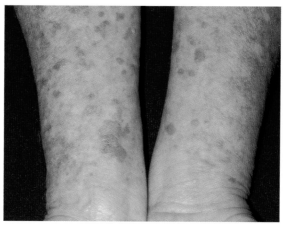

Figure 11.10. Lichen planus is an itchy skin condition of unknown origin that produces small, shiny, flat-topped, pink or purple raised spots. Image appears with permission from VisualDx © Logical Images, Inc.

Itch in lichen planus

Intense itch tends to affect most patients with lichen planus. The itchiest form of lichen planus is known as hypertrophic lichen planus, which most often occurs on the lower extremities (frequently on the shins) and presents as thick **plaques**.

Treatment for itch associated with lichen planus

High potency topical corticosteroids, tacrolimus, cyclosporine, topical retinoids, and UVB therapy are specific treatments for lichen planus that may be especially effective in reducing itch.

Did you know?

The skin condition lichen planus is often described by the six Ps: purple, polygonal, pruritic, planar (flat-topped), papules, and plaques.

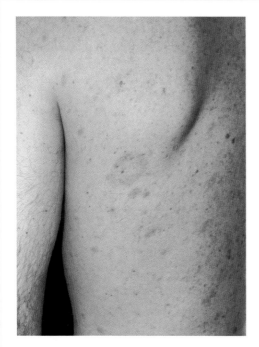

Figure 11.11. Pityriasis rosea is an itchy rash commonly found on the trunk that creates a pattern called a herald patch. Image appears with permission from VisualDx © Logical Images, Inc.

Additional Inflammatory Skin Conditions: Pityriasis Rosea

What is pityriasis rosea?

Pityriasis rosea is an acute, **self-limiting** skin rash that often begins with a single large lesion known as a *herald patch* (figure 11.11). Many times this initial herald patch can be misdiagnosed as eczema or psoriasis. However, the lesion is often followed one to two weeks later by a more widespread rash lasting for approximately six weeks.

What causes pityriasis rosea?

While the precise cause of pityriasis rosea is unknown, it is thought to be the result of an infectious process. Indeed, pityriasis rosea is often preceded by symptoms consistent with a viral upper respiratory infection. Pityriasis rosea has specifically been associated with human herpesvirus 7, though the extent of the association is unclear.

Itch in pityriasis rosea

Itch is a frequent complaint in a significant portion of patients with pityriasis rosea and can be severe in a subset of them.

Treatments for itch associated with pityriasis rosea

Oral antihistamines and topical corticosteroids are common treatments to relieve itch associated with pityriasis rosea. In severe cases oral corticosteroids can be used. Ultraviolet radiation exposure (whether through sunlight or artificial means) can also be used to reduce itch. Other topical over-the-counter remedies include calamine lotion.

Additional Inflammatory Skin Conditions: Pityriasis Lichenoides

Pityriasis lichenoides describes a diffuse rash similar to psoriasis in appearance that tends to affect adolescents and young adults. The rash has an undefined cause, though it has been associated with infections and autoimmunity. It has two forms: the more clinically severe form known as pityriasis lichenoides et varioliformis acuta (PLEVA; figure 11.12) and the chronic and more mild form known as pityriasis lichenoides chronica (PLC; figure 11.13). PLEVA is characterized by the sudden development of small, scaling **papules** that quickly blister and crust over within a few months. PLC, in contrast, is characterized by a slower, more gradual development of small, scaling papules that may last for a more extended time.

Itch in pityriasis lichenoides

Patients with PLEVA often experience intense itch (along with pain and tenderness), while itch is much less common in PLC.

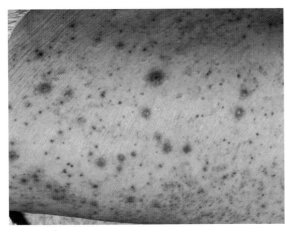

Figure 11.12. Pityriasis lichenoides et varioliformis acuta, a rare itchy skin rash with reddish brown **papules** that ulcerate and form open sores. Image appears with permission from VisualDx © Logical Images, Inc.

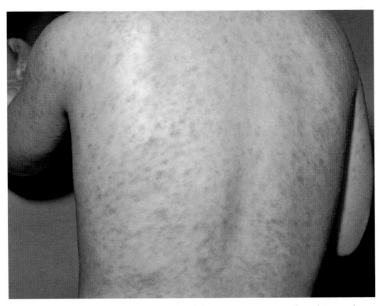

Figure 11.13. Pityriasis lichenoides chronica, a rare itchy skin rash with small scaling **papules,** is commonly found on the trunk and extremities. Image appears with permission from VisualDx © Logical Images, Inc.

Treatments for itch associated with pityriasis lichenoides

Treatments for itch can include ultraviolet radiation exposure (either through sunlight or artificial means) and topical corticosteroids. Other drugs that suppress the immune system, such as tacrolimus or pimecrolimus, may also have some efficacy. In more severe cases oral corticosteroids or methotrexate may be used.

Drug-Induced Pruritus

Several drugs may cause or exacerbate itch, including the following: aspirin (given to many patients with coronary artery disease), opioids (including a number of different medications given for chronic pain), angiotensin-converting-enzyme, or ACE, inhibitors (including several anti-hypertensive medications), and epidermal growth factor receptor (EGFR) inhibitors given for cancer.

Pruritus of Undetermined Origin

Some patients for whom the origin of their itching has not been discovered are given the diagnosis of "pruritus of undetermined origin."

Before this diagnosis is made, a careful evaluation should be made by your doctor to exclude both dermatologic and non-dermatologic causes of your pruritus. These include the following:

▶ Physical examination to evaluate for the presence of primary skin lesions (for example, lesions associated with atopic dermatitis, psoriasis, or cutaneous T-cell lymphoma).

▶ Systemic causes for pruritus should be excluded by performing the following laboratory tests:

  ▶ *Complete blood count (CBC).* This test looks at the different types of blood cells in the body (including red and white blood cells as well as platelets). An abnormality in these tests can alert the physician to hematologic abnormalities or clues about other types of underlying systemic disease.

- *Erythrocyte sedimentation rate (ESR).* This test is a good marker of the level of inflammation in the body.
- *Liver function tests (LFTs).* It is important to make sure that there are no abnormalities in the liver and the associated biliary system, since they can be a cause of itch.
- *Blood urea nitrogen / Creatinine.* All of these studies (if abnormal) can alert the physician to pathologies related to the kidney.
- *Thyroid function tests.* These studies can alert the physician to the presence of abnormal functioning of the thyroid gland. Hyperthyroidism is more commonly associated with chronic itch than is hypothyroidism.
- *Chest x-ray.* A chest x-ray may alert the physicians to underlying malignancies responsible for the chronic itch.

- The following tests may also be indicated, based on your physician's concerns and your medical history:
  - HIV serology
  - Stool studies for ova and parasites
  - Iron studies (to look for iron deficiency anemia, as it has been associated with chronic itch)
  - Computed tomography (CT) scan of the chest or abdomen when a lymphoma or other malignancy is suspected
  - Magnetic resonance imaging (MRI) of the spine in people who are suspected to have a neuropathic itch, particularly brachioradial pruritus and notalgia paresthetica

12

Psychogenic Itch

Itch is highly associated with the brain and mental processes. Researchers have found that simply thinking about itch or watching another person itching will cause you to scratch. This itch that results from thoughts or feelings is known as *psychogenic itch*.

Emotional stress can induce or aggravate itch. Indeed, there is an interrelationship between chronic stress, itch, and anxiety/depression (see figure 12.1). Another important factor is that chronic itch can lead to a lack of sleep, which can further decrease the threshold for anxiety and depressive symptoms.

A study found that patients with atopic dermatitis (see chapter 3) experienced more intense itch than usual while they watched videos of others scratching. An explanation for this finding could be that watching others scratching could cause people distress by bringing back memories of severe scratching episodes. The act of scratching has in turn been suggested as a way for people to provide temporary relief for their inner tensions. These examples illustrate the enhanced role psychological factors play in the perception of itch among people with especially itchy conditions such as atopic dermatitis and psoriasis. In addition, studies have

 See jhupress.com/livingwithitch/ for a video showing contagious itch.

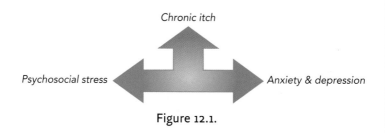

Chronic itch

Psychosocial stress

Anxiety & depression

Figure 12.1.

shown that people with atopic dermatitis have a significantly greater level of anxiety, depression, and even thoughts of suicide.

In particular, depression has been found to correlate with the intensity of itch in people suffering from atopic dermatitis, chronic urticaria (see chapter 6), and psoriasis (see chapter 4). Studies have also shown that people with depression can suffer severe itch that often responds to common antidepressant medications including tricyclic antidepressants (TCAs), noradrenergic selective serotoninergic antidepressants (NaSSA), and selective serotonin reuptake inhibitors (SSRIs). Mirtazapine, an NaSSA, may be particularly effective, as it has been shown to significantly reduce itch (especially nighttime itch) and to decrease both anxiety and depressive symptoms. Similar to people who have depression, people who have fibromyalgia (a common syndrome with depressive symptoms, widespread pain, and lack of sleep) may also have chronic itch.

While the exact mechanism behind itch of psychogenic origin is unknown, it is likely that an alteration in chemicals in the brain, such as neurotransmitters (for example, serotonin, acetylcholine, epinephrine, and dopamine) and naturally occurring opioids, plays a significant role. Below we will discuss specific diseases that can cause psychogenic itch.

Psychogenic pruritus is diagnosed by clinicians when no skin

Did you know?

The skin and the brain both originate from the same precursor cell layer termed the *embryonic neuroectoderm*.

pathology or underlying medical disease can be identified but when severe itch is experienced. People with psychogenic pruritus may have associated psychiatric disorders or may recently have experienced significant events in their lives causing psychological distress. These people have significant amounts of skin **excoriation** and thickening of the skin known as **lichenification**. They may significantly benefit from psychoactive drugs, including antidepressants, as well as from psychotherapy.

One rare cause of psychogenic itch is called delusion of *parasitosis*. In this disorder, people have a strong belief that they are infected by parasites, but close clinical examination by physicians does not reveal evidence to support this assertion. These people are often treated with antipsychotic medications such as pimozide and olanzapine.

People who have obsessive-compulsive disorder may experience localized itch (a classic example is anogenital pruritus and **trichotillomania)**. A common treatment for these conditions is antidepressants and psychological therapies such as cognitive-behavioral therapy.

When talking about psychosocial issues, it is important to also mention how poor social support affects skin diseases. Studies have shown a clear inverse relationship between the amount of social support people have and the intensity of itch that they experience; in other words, people who have better social support experience less severe itch. An explanation for this finding may simply be that increased social support can significantly reduce the amount of stress people experience in their life.

See jhupress.com/livingwithitch/ for an interactive graphic on how itch can come from damage along any point of the nervous system and brain.

From a treatment standpoint, it is clear that to manage itch, relevant **psychosomatic** factors must be addressed. In addition to making itch worse, anxiety and depression can affect people's cognitive outlook toward disease and negatively impact treatment outcomes.

In addition to the pharmacologic treatments mentioned above, several non-pharmacologic therapeutic strategies may also be helpful, including biofeedback, cognitive-behavioral therapy, mediation, psychotherapy, and relaxation training. In Europe, there are also established schools for eczema (called, fittingly, eczema schools) and itch reduction where family members and patients participate alongside one another in group sessions to discuss coping mechanisms to reduce itch.

PART III

Treating Itch

13
Preventing Itch without Medications

Moisturizers

Moisturizers (also including barrier creams and emollients) are over-the-counter agents whose application should be an important part of the daily regimen for people suffering from chronic itch. Moisturizers are composed of mixtures of chemical agents (including artificial or natural oils) that help make skin softer by increasing its water content. Moisturizers include three broad classes: ointments, creams, and lotions.

▶ *Ointments* are approximately 80% oil and 20% water. Ointments are excellent at keeping the skin moisturized, but they are often avoided because they are greasy.

▶ *Creams* are less greasy than ointments and are composed of approximately 50% oil and 50% water.

▶ *Lotions* are the least thick formulation, with an even greater component of water than oil. Lotions are often not as effective as creams and ointments because their greater water component tends to quickly evaporate.

Using moisturizers to treat dry skin and damage to the skin barrier is very important in preventing itch. Many studies have shown that dry skin can cause or significantly worsen itch.

Moisturizers are effective in reducing itch through preventing water loss from the skin (known as *transepidermal water loss*). To highlight the importance of preventing water loss from the skin, a study found that the degree of transepidermal water loss is associated with itch intensity in people with atopic dermatitis (see chapter 3). One explanation for this finding may be that a decreased skin barrier may expose nerve endings to common irritants.

To help keep as much water in the skin as possible, moisturizing agents should be applied directly to the skin as soon as possible after bathing (ideally within minutes) and can be applied several times a day.

Bathing

A few points are important to keep in mind during bathing:

▶ Use a non-irritating cleanser.

▶ Avoid soaps, because they tend to have a high pH.

▶ When choosing cleansers and moisturizers, opt for low pH cleansers, and moisturizers (less than a pH of 6). The reason for this is because the skin, particularly the outer surface known as the *stratum corneum*, is acidic in nature, with an average pH of 4.5 to 6 (acidic compounds correspond to a lower pH, while more basic compounds have a higher pH). Many of the soaps that are currently available have an average pH—a pH higher than 9. One mechanism for greater itch associated with a higher pH is the increased activity of **proteases** in the skin (see chapter 3).

▶ Examples of brands of cleansers known to have a healthier, more acidic pH include Cetaphil, Sebamed, and Vanicream.

▶ Patting the skin dry with a towel is preferred. Do not scrub the skin harshly with a towel after showering or bathing. This may irritate the skin and cause increased water loss.

▶ After taking a shower or bath, apply any prescription medications (such as topical corticosteroids) to your skin before applying moisturizers.

Oatmeal Bath

While a traditional water bath is sufficient, some "specialty baths" may also be helpful. One of these baths is an oatmeal bath. This can be made by using fine plain, unflavored oatmeal. You can grind the oatmeal into small pieces using a spoon. You should add about a quarter to three-quarters of a cup of oatmeal to a full bathtub of water. Alternatively, there are also some baths containing oatmeal that are already made, such as the Aveeno "soothing bath treatment," which is made of 100% pure oatmeal. You can have these baths as often as once a day. Oatmeal functions to soothe irritated skin. Some studies have shown that oatmeal contains anti-inflammatory mediators that reduce inflammation of the skin.

Itch-Reducing Garments

Wool and certain artificial fibers can irritate the skin, activate nerve fibers, and induce itch. With this in mind, new garments have been developed that have less friction and form a protective layer around the skin. These garments help to block outside signals that trigger nerve fibers in the skin (including irritating clothing and sweat).

Additional Tips

▶ Keep fingernails cut short to reduce the effects of scratching.

▶ Try to stay in a cool environment. Itch can be exacerbated by warmer temperatures.

▶ Along these lines, you can see if you have better relief of your itch when you use moisturizers that were kept in the refrigerator.

▶ Avoid skin irritants. Avoid clothing made of artificial fibers or wool, and avoid irritating cleansers.

▶ Try to wear light clothing made of cotton.

▶ If there is a specific area of the body that is itchy, you can try to occlude (cover) the area with a moisturizer and occlude the moisturizer with a dressing on top to keep you from scratching the itchy area.

▶ A humidifier may help people during the winter who are more prone to dry skin.

▶ Extreme changes from high to low humidity may aggravate itch. Avoid dramatic changes in humidity.

▶ Try to avoid extreme changes of temperature (at either end of the spectrum).

▶ Instead of scratching lesions directly, try patting them (will help minimize direct skin injury).

14

Topical Treatments for Itch

Topical therapies—those applied directly to the skin or other external part of the body—are usually most effective in people who have itch that is localized to certain regions. The various topical agents are listed in table 14.1.

Topical Corticosteroids

Topical corticosteroids are anti-inflammatory creams and ointments that are often the first agents prescribed by dermatologists for people suffering from itch associated with inflamma-

Table 14.1. Commonly prescribed corticosteroids

Potency class	Corticosteroids
I (ultrahigh)	Clobetasol proprionate 0.05%
II (high)	Betamethasone valerate 0.1%
III (medium/moderate)	Triamcinolone acetonide 0.1% Mometasone furoate 0.1%
IV (mild)	Hydrocortisone 0.5–2.5%

Note: Prolonged use of topical corticosteroids could cause skin thinning and swelling of blood vessels in the skin. Mild topical steroids are recommended to be used in thin skin areas, such as the face, and sensitive areas, such as on the armpits and groin (especially areas under occlusion).

tory skin diseases such as atopic dermatitis, psoriasis, contact dermatitis, and lichen planus (see chapter 11). Topical corticosteroids are meant to serve as treatments specifically directed at the inflammation as opposed to treating the underlying cause of itch. Specifically, topical corticosteroids do not directly decrease itch, but rather indirectly decrease the sensation of itch by reducing inflammation of the skin. If there no inflammation present (which appears as a rash), then the efficacy of these medications is of limited value. Caution should be used when applying topical corticosteroids to certain parts of the body (figure 14.1).

Topical corticosteroids come in several different potencies and vehicles (including creams, ointments, gels, and lotions). Table 14.2 shows one way to classify topical corticosteroids by their potency and lists the names of a few commonly prescribed steroids in the different classes.

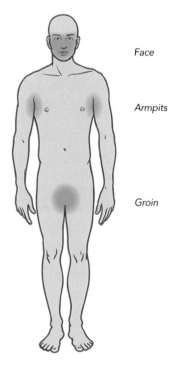

Face

Armpits

Groin

Figure 14.1. Places to use caution when applying high potency topical corticosteroids

Table 14.2. Topical anti-itch treatments

Pharmaceutical agent	Common doses used	Examples of brand names containing these compounds	Conditions where this agent may be especially helpful	Side effects
OVER-THE-COUNTER TOPICAL ANTI-ITCH AGENTS				
Hydrocortisone	1%	Cortizone, Cortaid Preparation H	Inflammatory conditions of the skin	Skin thinning, swelling of blood vessels
Menthol	1–7% cream	Sarna, Bengay	Patients whose itch responds well to the application of an ice cube or to cold showers	Skin irritation (including hypersensitivity and burns) may occur with higher concentrations
Pramoxine	1–2.5%	Sarna sensitive	Facial eczema, atopic eczema, itch associated with dry skin (aka xerosis), particularly for itch associated with the face and genital areas, uremic pruritus, and neuropathic itch	Skin irritation and dryness at the affected area
Strontium chloride	4%	TriCalm	Neuropathic itch, itch associated with scars	Possible mild irritation
Capsaicin	0.025–0.1% cream	Zostrix, Capzasin	Different forms of neuropathic itch, atopic dermatitis, psoriasis, and itch associated with chronic kidney disease	Transient burning sensation upon application (this is often only temporary for the first few applications)

continued

Table 14.2. Topical anti-itch treatments (continued)

Pharmaceutical agent	Common doses used	Examples of brand names containing these compounds	Conditions where this agent may be especially helpful	Side effects
Camphor	0.45%	Benadryl anti-itch gel	Sunburn, poison ivy, eczema	Skin irritation (can worsen itch in some people)
Calamine	7.5%	Aveeno anti-itch cream	Sunburn, poison ivy, eczema	Not known to irritate the skin
Salicylic acid	2–6%	Salex 6%	Lichen simplex chronicus	Stinging sensation
N-palmitoylethanolamine		Mimyx	Atopic dematitis and itch associated with chronic kidney disease	
TOPICAL ANTI-ITCH AGENTS NEEDING A PRESCRIPTION FROM YOUR DOCTOR				
Topical corticosteroids (available in several different potencies)	See table 14.1	See table 14.1	Atopic dermatitis, psoriasis (among many others)	Skin thinning, swelling of blood vessels, suppression of body's natural adrenaline (rare and in severe cases)

Generic name	Brand name	Concentration	Indications	Side effects
Doxepin	Zonalon	5%	Psoriasis, atopic dermatitis	Drowsiness and localized burning sensations (should be avoided in children)
Pimecrolimus	Elidel	1% cream	Atopic dermatitis, contact dermatitis, and particularly for facial, hand, and anogenital itch	Transient stinging/burning sensations
Tacrolimus	Protopic	0.03–0.1% ointment	Atopic dermatitis, contact dermatitis, and particularly for facial, hand, and anogenital itch	Transient stinging/ burning sensations
Lidocaine (topical anesthetic)	EMLA (combination of lidocaine and prilocaine)	2.5–5%	Anal pruritus, neuropathic itch (notalgia paresthetica, brachioradial pruritus), postburn itch	Methemoglobinemia
Prilocaine (topical anesthetic)	EMLA (combination of lidocaine and prilocaine)	2.5%	Anal pruritus, notalgia paresthetica, postburn pruritus	Methemoglobinemia
Polidocanol	Balneum Hermal Plus	3% (polidocanol is often formulated with 5% urea)	Atopic dermatitis, contact dermatitis, psoriasis	Allergic contact dermatitis

Source: Adapted from "Pathophysiology and Clinical Aspects of Pruritus" in Fitzpatrick's Dermatology in General Medicine, 8th ed., pp. 1147–1158. Eds. Goldsmith LA, Katz SI, Gilchrest BA, Paller AS, Lefell DJ, Wolff K. McGraw Hill Medical, NY.

See jhupress.com/livingwithitch/ for a video showing how to apply topical medications for itch.

Wet Pajamas

Wet-wrap treatments are an extremely important tool in managing severe atopic dermatitis (especially for acute flares), psoriasis, and in a number of other pruritic disorders. Just one week's treatment can lead to a significant improvement in the itch that people experience.

Wet wraps work the following ways: softening the skin by increasing moisture, preventing water loss through the skin, cooling the skin, providing occlusion (which can enhance the absorption of medications), and providing a physical barrier to prevent scratching.

Double layer wet pajamas are worn during the night but can be an effective method to reduce itch during all times of the day.

 See jhupress.com/livingwithitch/ for a video on the double wet layer pajama treatment for relief of chronic itch.

The basic technique for double wet layers pajamas is as follows:

1. Take a shower or soak yourself in a bath.

2. A moisturizing lotion, cream, or topical corticosteroid should be applied to the affected areas of the skin.

3. A wet pair of pajamas that has been soaked in water should be worn on top of the creams.

4. A dry pair of pajamas should be worn on top.

5. Now you are ready to go to sleep. You should sleep through the night. If for some reason your itch is aggravated, you can remove the dry layer of pajamas and re-wet the inner layer.

Wet layer pajamas are recommended to be used in one week intervals.

People often struggle determining how much topical corticosteroid to apply to the body. While the answer to this question is complex and based on the extent of disease and the potency of the corticosteroid, generally, when using a mild to medium topical corticosteroid, use the fingertip rule. Here is how you can use the index finger to estimate the amount of topical corticosteroid to use on the body:

▶ The front and back of the trunk each require approximately six or seven fingertip amounts of corticosteroid.

▶ The hand requires approximately one fingertip.

▶ The face, neck, and ears together require approximately two fingertip units.

Cooling Agents

Menthol has been used for centuries to treat itch. Topical menthol is effective at reducing itch through a cooling effect on the skin. It may work through activating nerve fibers that transmit a cooling sensation or through specific transient receptor potential (TRP) channels (see chapter 2) on nerve fibers and **keratinocytes**. Menthol has also been reported to work on the kappa-**opioid receptor** system.

This medication is helpful in people with itch that is improved with a cold shower or the application of an ice cube (for example, people with neuropathic itch including brachioradial pruritus and notalgia paresthetica; see chapter 7).

Other cooling agents that are available (and are often combined with other antipruritic therapies) include camphor and calamine lotion.

Capsaicin

Topical capsaicin (the active ingredient of chili peppers) releases a molecule in the nervous system known as *Substance P*. Exactly how capsaicin works at suppressing itch is not fully

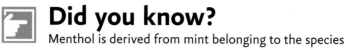

Did you know?

Menthol is derived from mint belonging to the species *Mentha arvensis*.

understood, but it is known that exposure to capsaicin can deplete Substance P. Capsaicin also is known to work through the *transient receptor potential vanilloid receptor-1* (TRPV1) (see chapter 2). Initial application of capsaicin causes a transient burning sensation. However, this adverse effect typically resolves after this medicine is used for a few days or if it is used alongside a topical anesthetic.

Capsaicin is especially effective at reducing itch that originates from nerve fibers (neuropathic itch) including postherpetic itch, brachioradial pruritus, and notalgia paresthetica (see chapter 7). In addition, capsaicin is effective at reducing itch associated with atopic dermatitis, psoriasis, and chronic kidney disease. Caution should be used: avoid applying capsaicin to genital and mucosal areas, as it causes a stinging sensation.

Topical Anesthetics

Topical anesthetics that have been found to have anti-itch effects include pramoxine, prilocaine, lidocaine, and polidocanol. These agents work by blocking the transmission of nerve impulses. Pramoxine 1% is effective in treating many different types of itch. In particular, it is effective at reducing itch in facial and genital areas, as well as treating neuropathic itch. In addition, a pramoxine-based anti-itch lotion has shown efficacy in treating pruritus in adults who are undergoing hemodialysis. Polidocanol is another topical agent available that is not currently available in the United States. A combination of 3% Polidocanol and 5% urea significantly reduced itch in people with atopic dermatitis, contact dermatitis, and psoriasis.

Strontium Gel

A moisturizer containing strontium hydrochloride 4% gel (TriCalm) was found to reduce itch of different types including neuropathic itch, itch associated with a type of scar tissue called a keloid, and itch caused by histamine. Although its exact mechanism of action is unclear, it seems to work on **ion channels** in nerve fibers that transmit itch and pain in the skin.

Tacrolimus and Pimecrolimus

These are two non-steroid-based anti-inflammatory medications known as *calcineurin inhibitors* (brand names Elidel and Protopic). These drugs are immunomodulating agents, meaning that they work similarly to corticosteroids in suppressing inflammation. On the molecular level, these drugs are thought to work on TRPV1 (see chapter 2). These drugs have been effective in reducing itch associated with atopic dermatitis and are also typically used for facial, hand, and anogenital itch. These agents are particularly useful for the face and armpits (figure 14.1), areas where topical corticosteroids are traditionally not used due to concern for skin **atrophy**. A commonly encountered side effect from these drugs is a temporary burning or stinging sensation.

Doxepin

The antidepressant Doxepin is a potent antihistamine as well as a sedative. In particular, Doxepin 5% cream is effective at reducing itch in people with atopic dermatitis (among other conditions). Doxepin cream can also be absorbed systemically by the body and lead to a significant amount of drowsiness.

Topical Cannabinoids

The rationale for using topical **cannabinoids** in the treatment of itch came with the finding that cannabinoid **receptors** are expressed on **keratinocytes**, **mast cells**, and nerve fibers. N-palmitoylethanolamine is a medication that stimulates cannabinoid receptors. It has been incorporated into creams and has been shown to reduce itch associated with atopic dermatitis and chronic kidney disease.

Topical Salicylates

Topical salicylic acid (aspirin) is an effective keratolytic agent, which means it is effective at reducing thickening of the skin (which can occur as a result of chronic scratching). Topical salicylates have been shown to be effective in lichen simplex chronicus—a form of itch that is localized and associated with thickened skin. Salicylic acid softens the skin through increasing hydration. Salicylic acid also inhibits prostaglandins, which are lipids that can sensitize nerve fibers to itchy stimuli.

15

Systemic Treatments for Itch

Systemic treatments for itch use medications that travel through the bloodstream and reach the skin and nerves all over the body.

 See jhupress.com/livingwithitch/ for an interactive graphic on medications that work on skin, nerves, spinal cord, and brain.

Antihistamines

Oral antihistamines have long been one of the first-line treatments for itch. As their name suggests, antihistamines work through blocking the action of histamine. Thus, antihistamines can be effective in disorders where histamine is what triggers itch (for example chronic urticaria, or hives).

There are several types of antihistamines, which can be divided into sedating and non-sedating (see table 15.1). Sedating antihistamines, on the one hand, such as hydroxyzine, may be particularly useful for itch that is most severe at night. On the other hand, non-sedating antihistamines, such as cetirizine, desloratadine, loratadine, and levocetirizine, may be more helpful for daytime itch and are especially useful at targeting diseases where histamine is an important component of the itch (for example urticaria, drug-related itch, and chronic insect bites). Non-sedating antihistamines are of limited efficacy in other chronic types of itch. Table 15.2 shows the various systemic treatments for itch.

Antidepressants

In chapter 12, we discussed the interrelationship between itch, the brain, and the psyche. This connection explains why antidepressants have been shown to be effective in reducing itch in many people. It is important to note that all antidepressants usually take about two to four weeks to get into a person's system before a significant benefit can be seen. Antidepressants can be generally classified into two categories based on whether they increase the amount of the neurotransmitter serotonin alone or the amount of both serotonin and norepinephrine in the brain.

1. *Antidepressants that increase the amount of norepinephrine and serotonin in the brain.* Mirtazapine increases the amount of both norepinephrine and serotonin in the brain. For patients with chronic itch, Mirtazapine may be an especially effective drug since it can improve mood and enhance sleep. One of the side

Table 15.1. Antihistamines (sedating and non-sedating types)

Type	Example
Sedating antihistamines, known as first-generation antihistamines. These medications cross the blood-brain barrier (which is one reason they are so sedating).	Hydroxyzine Diphenhydramine (Benadryl) Chlorpheniramine maleate
Non-sedating antihistamines. These include both second- and third-generation antihistamines.	Second-generation antihistamines. These agents are longer-acting, have a slower onset of action, and in general are less sedating than first-generation antihistamines. Examples include cetirizine and loratadine. Third-generation antihistamines. These agents are very similar to second-generation antihistamines, but with slightly increased efficacy and fewer adverse drug reactions. Examples include fexofenadine, levocetirizine, and desloratadine.

Table 15.2. Systemic treatments for pruritus

Medication class	Medication and dosages	Main indication	Major side effect
Antihistamines (first generation)	Hydroxyzine Adults: 25–100 mg/day in three divided doses Children 30 months to 15 years: 1 mg/kg/day in divided doses Diphenhydramine Adults: 25–50 mg twice a day Children >2 years old: 1–2 mg/kg every 6–8 hours Chlorpheniramine maleate Adults: 4 mg every 6–8 hours Children: 0.1 mg/kg every 6–8 hours	Nocturnal itch (therefore are usually given only at night)	Sedation
Antihistamines (second generation)	Loratadine Adults and children ≥12 years: 10 mg a day Children 2–12 years: >30 kg:10 mg a day; ≤30 kg: 5 mg a day Cetirizine Adults and children ≥6 years: 10 mg a day or 5 mg twice a day Children 2–5 yrs: 2.5 mg twice a day or 5 mg a day Renal or hepatic insufficiency: reduce dosages by half Fexofenadine Adults and children ≥12 years: 60 mg twice a day or 120 mg a day or 180 mg a day Children 6–11 years: 30 mg twice a day Renal impairment: consider lower dose of 60 mg a day	Urticaria Mastocytosis Insect bite reactions	Infrequent: Drowsiness Dry mouth

continued

Table 15.2. Systemic treatments for pruritus (continued)

Medication class	Medication and dosages	Main indication	Major side effect
Anticonvulsants	Gabapentin 300–3600 mg/day in three divided doses In dialysis patients, 100–300 mg after each dialysis Pregabalin 150–450mg/day in two divided doses	Neuropathic itch Uremic pruritus Prurigo nodularis Post-burn pruritus	Drowsiness Dizziness Leg swelling Constipation or diarrhea Blurred vision
Mu-opioid receptor antagonists	Naltrexone 25–50 mg each morning	Pruritus associated with cholestasis, atopic dermatitis, and chronic urticaria	Nausea and vomiting Sleepiness Reversal of opioid analgesia Liver toxicity rarely
Kappa-opioid receptor agonists	Butorphanol 1–4 mg intranasally each night Nalfurafine 2.5–5μg	Uremic pruritus (nalfurafine)	Butorphanol: Drowsiness Nausea and vomiting Nalfurafine: Insomnia
Antidepressants	Mirtazapine 7.5–15 mg each night initially, up to 45 mg each night SSRIs Paroxetine, 10–40 mg a day Sertraline, 75–100 mg a day	Malignancy-associated pruritus Nocturnal pruritus in atopic dermatitis Consider in pruritus associated with depression and/or anxiety	Mirtazapine: Drowsiness Weight gain SSRIs: Drowsiness Sleepiness Sexual dysfunction

Antidepressants (cont'd)	Fluvoxamine, 25 mg for 3 days, then 50–150 mg a day Tricyclic antidepressants Doxepin, 10–100 mg each night Amitriptyline, 25–75 mg each night	Pruritus associated with hematological malignancies and solid tumors (paroxetine) Cholestatic pruritus (sertraline) Chronic idiopathic urticaria (doxepin) Neuropathic itch (amitriptyline)	Anti-cholinergic effects Drowsiness Dry eyes and mouth Blurred vision Urinary retention Cardiovascular effects Blood pressure can fall suddenly when standing Conduction disturbances
Thalidomide	100 mg a day	Prurigo nodularis Uremic pruritus	Birth defects Peripheral neuropathy Drowsiness
Neurokinin-1 receptor antagonist	Aprepitant 80 mg a day	Hematological malignancies Solid tumors Prurigo nodularis	Nausea Dizziness
Phototherapy	UVB, broad and narrowband UVA Combined UVA and UVB PUVA, oral and topical	Atopic dermatitis Psoriasis Uremic pruritus	Tanning Skin malignancies

Source: Adapted from Tey HL, Yosipovitch G, Bernhard HD. "Pruritus." American College of Physicians.

effects of Mirtazapine is that it may stimulate your appetite (and cause weight gain); another side effect is drowsiness.

2. *Antidepressants that increase the amount of serotonin in the brain (aka selective serotonin reuptake inhibitors, or SSRIs).* These drugs specifically increase primarily the amount of serotonin in the brain and include fluoxetine (Prozac), fluvoxamine, paroxetine and sertraline.

Neuroactive Medications

These **neuroactive** medications (also known as anticonvulsants), which include gabapentin and pregabalin, work on the central nervous system. In addition to controlling itch, these medications have also been shown to be effective at controlling pain in people with chronic pain syndromes. While how they work isn't precisely known, they are thought to decrease the processing of itchy stimuli through the nerves to the brain. Since they are thought to act on nerve fibers, they are especially effective in forms of neuropathic itch (see chapter 7), such as postherpetic neuropathic itch, brachioradial pruritus, and notalgia paresthetica, where the onset of itch is specifically tied to nerve fibers. In addition, these medications have been shown to be effective in people suffering from cutaneous lymphomas and in people with chronic kidney disease (when used after each dialysis session). Gabapentin should be avoided in people with itch resulting from liver disease, as it may aggravate itch in these people. Some common side effects of **neuroactive** drugs include drowsiness, gait imbalances, blurry vision, and constipation.

Opioid Stimulators and Blockers

Opioids, such as morphine, have been known for some time to be extremely important in blocking pain transmission; they have also been shown to worsen itch. Recently, imbalances in opioids naturally found in the body have been implicated in the pathophysiology of itch. Recent research has revealed the importance of subgroups of **opioid receptors** in the brain, including mu and kappa opioids. Specifically, there seems to be an inverse relation-

Morphine and other common opioid medications reduce pain, while conversely having the potential effect of exacerbating itch. This itch is caused by stimulation of the mu-opioid receptors, which are located in the brain and various organs. These receptors can be blocked by mu-opioid receptor blockers, such as naltrexone.

ship present: stimulation of the mu-opioid receptor increases itch and stimulation of the kappa-opioid receptor decreases itch.

Mu-opioid receptor blockers

These blockers include naltrexone and nalmfene. Naltrexone (which is more commonly prescribed) has been shown to reduce itch in people with liver disease, chronic kidney disease, atopic dermatitis, and those suffering from post-burn itch.

Kappa-opioid receptor stimulators

Agents that stimulate the κ-opioid receptor include butorphanol and nalfurafine. Butorphanol (a medication also shown to have promise in the treatment of chronic migraine headaches) both stimulates and blocks the opioid receptors. It can be given intranasally and can be effective in the treatment of chronic refractory itch in people whose itch is the result of inflammatory skin diseases and systemic conditions. It is important to note that this is one of the last-line treatments for itch and is considered a controlled substance by the FDA. Nalfurafine has been shown to be effective in treating itch in people with chronic kidney disease (it is already approved for this use in Japan).

Drugs That Work on the Immune System
Oral corticosteroids

These are drugs that reduce the amount of inflammation present in the body. They have no direct anti-itch effect. They are particularly effective for itchy conditions associated with skin diseases with rash that is not infectious. Prolonged use of these medications is not recommended due to adverse side effects. In only a few skin diseases, such as pemphigus and dermatomyositis, a prolonged use of these medications for a year is required to control the disease.

Immunosuppressants: Cyclosporine, azathioprine, and mycophenolate mofetil

These drugs are effective at suppressing an overactive immune system. These agents can have efficacy in controlling itch associated with atopic dermatitis, since this disease often features an overactive immune system. These agents are recommended for short-term use in the treatment of atopic dermatitis in people whose symptoms have failed to respond to other, more conventional, therapies. People also need appropriate monitoring when taking these agents. People on azathioprine should also have lab work done regularly to check blood counts and liver enzymes for abnormalities. In addition, cyclosporine has been associated with high blood pressure and kidney dysfunction and requires careful monthly monitoring of kidney function, while people taking mycophenolate mofetil may experience diarrhea and nausea.

Methotrexate

Methotrexate is an oral anticancer drug that can also be used to suppress the immune system in low doses in people who have atopic dermatitis. This drug interacts with the immune system by inhibiting DNA synthesis. Methotrexate can be an effective drug in the treatment of eczema (see chapter 3), psoriasis (see chapter 4), and cutaneous T-cell lymphoma (see chapter 5). In some patients, this drug lowers the white blood cell count, especially in the first weeks after it is given. A low white blood cell count increases the chance of getting a serious infection. This drug can also cause liver toxicity, especially in those who drink alcohol regularly or have a fatty liver. Therefore regular monitoring of blood counts and liver function is required when patients are taking methotrexate.

Thalidomide

Thalidomide is an oral agent that has the effect of decreasing the overactivity of the immune and nervous systems. It should be one of the last-line treatments for itch associated with chronic kidney disease, priugo nodularis (a skin disease that produces itchy nodules on the arms and legs), or cutaneous T-cell lymphoma. Thalidomide has significant potential side effects, especially birth defects in offspring of women of childbearing age (it is not to be used at all during pregnancy), peripheral nerve fiber damage, and drowsiness. It is given by dermatologists who have a special license to administer this drug and requires monthly visits to monitor its side effects.

Dapsone

This is an antibacterial agent that also has a significant anti-inflammatory effect. Its anti-inflammatory (and likely antipruritic) effect comes from its blocking myeloperoxidase, a protein that is expressed in neutrophils, which is a type of inflammatory cell predominant in skin lesions in people who have dermatitis herpetiformis. Dapsone may also be effective in the treatment of itch in people with bullous pemphigoid and urticaria (hives).

Aprepitant

Aprepitant is the only FDA-approved blocker of the **neurokinin 1 receptor**, which binds Substance P (a neurotransmitter and inflammatory chemical known to be involved in itch transmission). While large studies are lacking, in small groups of people this agent has been shown to be effective in reducing itch associated with cutaneous T-cell lymphoma (in particular for people with Sézary syndrome; see chapter 5), atopic dermatitis, solid tumors, chronic refractory itch, and itch associated with the use of epidermal growth factor receptor, which are anticancer drugs. This agent tends to be more expensive, and its efficacy as an antipruritic agent requires more investigation.

Phototherapy

Phototherapy can be helpful in the treatment of many itchy conditions (ranging from common dermatologic conditions such as atopic dermatitis and psoriasis to itch associated with systemic conditions including chronic kidney or liver disease and itch associated with HIV). The different forms of phototherapy include both broad-band and narrow-band ultraviolet B (UVB) and ultraviolet A (UVA). These agents can be used individually, in combination with one another, or with a compound known as psoralen that can be ingested orally or applied topically. While the exact mechanism is unknown for how phototherapy can decrease itch, it has been suggested that it results in the chemical modification of itch-producing factors.

A Psychological Approach

The brain is a key component in the itch transmission pathway. In addition, as described previously, psychological factors (including stress and anxiety) are extremely important factors in chronic itch. For this reason, psychological therapy has emerged as an important complement to pharmacologic therapy in the multidimensional treatment of chronic itch. Cognitive-behavioral therapies are important in helping people cope with their disease. Many people with chronic itch also have depression and anxiety, and treating these conditions can also improve the person's underlying itch. A previous study has shown that people with atopic dermatitis who received cognitive-behavioral therapy and relaxation training exhibited a substantial reduction in their itch a year later.

Alternative Therapies

The term *alternative therapy* in general is used to describe any medical treatment or intervention that has not been sufficiently scientifically documented or identified as safe and effective for a specific condition. Alternative therapy encompasses a variety of disciplines including acupuncture, relaxation techniques, guided

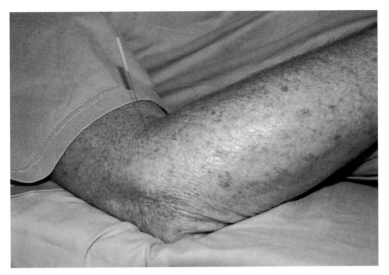

Figure 15.1. Acupuncture point for itch: Chinese medicine believes there is a distribution network that relates to internal organs called the Meridian System. The large intestine meridian L11 in the elbow was found to be an effective site for treating itch. Courtesy of Boyd Bailey.

imagery, yoga, hypnosis, biofeedback, aromatherapy, herbal remedies, massage therapy, and many others.

In the past decade, strong evidence has been accumulated regarding the benefits of mind-body therapies, such as acupuncture (figure 15.1), and some nutritional supplements for treating itch. Other alternative therapies such as therapeutic touch and dietary approaches have the potential to alleviate chronic itch in some cases. However, the evidence supporting these therapies is less concrete and is still emerging.

Conclusion

Chronic itch affects millions of people worldwide and comes in many different shapes and forms. There have recently been significant advances in our understanding of the mechanisms responsible for itch transmission. It is our hope that this understanding will lead to significant advancements in the treatment of this often-devastating condition. While there is currently no "simple recipe" available for treating chronic itch, there are many things people can do right now. It is our intention that this book provides useful information for itch sufferers along with their families and friends to better understand this debilitating condition. We hope that the personal stories of those coping with itch let people know they are not alone in their struggle against itch. We also hope these stories serve as examples of how important it is to have good communication about your condition with your doctors.

Our final statement for the many people that are suffering from chronic itch is simple: have hope and work to give yourself the knowledge to better understand and manage your condition.

atrophy: A decrease in size of a body organ, for example, skin.

cannabinoid: Any of various chemical constituents of cannabis or marijuana. The skin has receptors to some of these chemicals that can inhibit itch.

carcinoma, basal cell and squamous cell: Two types of common skin cancers. Basal is slow growing and the most common form of skin cancer. It rarely spreads to other organs. Squamous cell carcinoma is more aggressive and can spread to other organs.

ceramide: A lipid made up of a fatty acid and located within the membrane of cells. These cells can be found on the surface of the upper layers of the skin. Artificial ceramides are used as moisturizers in skin-care preparations.

cytokines: Chemicals made by the cells that act on other cells to stimulate or inhibit their function. They have a role in itch when skin is inflamed.

erosion: A shallow or superficial ulceration of the skin.

excoriation: A superficial loss of skin, produced by scratching.

ion channel: A part of the cell membrane that only allows certain ions, such as calcium, sodium, or potassium, to pass through it.

keloid: A sharply elevated, enlarging scar.

keratinocyte: The most common type of skin cells found in the epidermis. They make keratin, a protein that strengthens skin, hair, and nails.

lichenification: Thickening and hardening of the skin associated with repeated scratching.

mast cell: A cell found in skin during allergic reactions. When this type of cell is injured, it releases strong chemicals, including histamine and **proteases** that cause itch.

neuroactive: Something that stimulates neural, or brain, tissue.

neurokinin: A chemical known as a neuropeptide that is able to excite nerve cells.

opioid receptor: A protein that binds opium-like compounds in the brain and nervous system. These **receptors** are involved with both the beneficial effect of painkillers and the negative effects of opioids, including addictions. The three major types of these receptors are delta, kappa, and mu. Kappa receptors are known to inhibit itch. Mu opioids are among the most effective types of painkillers.

papule: A solid, rounded growth that is elevated from the skin up to 0.5 cm in diameter.

plaque: A well-circumscribed, elevated, superficial, solid lesion, greater than 1 cm in diameter.

proteases: Enzymes that hydrolyze proteins, or break them down to their component amino acids. Some of these enzymes bind to receptors and cause itch.

psychosomatic: A disorder having physical symptoms but originating from mental or emotional causes.

receptor: A specialized structure on the surface or interior of s cell that responds to chemical signals.

self-limiting: A condition that runs its course without the need of any medical treatment.

trichotillomania: The compulsion to tear or pluck out the hair on one's own head.

REFERENCES

Tey HL, Yosipovitch G, Bernhard JD. "Pruritus." American College of Physicians.

Valdes-Rodriguez R, Kwatra SG, Yosipovitch G. "Itch in Psoriasis: From Basic Mechanisms to Practical Treatments" *Psoriasis Forum* 2012; 18, no. 3.

Weisshaar E, Szepietowski JC, Darsow U, et al., "European Guideline on Chronic Pruritus,"*Acta Dermato-Venereologica* 2012; 92: 563-581.

Yosipovitch G, Bernhard JD, "Chronic Pruritus," *New England Journal Medicine* 2013; 368:1625-1634.

Yosipovitch G, Patel T, "Pathophysiology and Clinical Aspects of Pruritus" in, Goldsmith LA, Katz SI, Gilchrest BA, Paller AS, Lefell DJ, Wolff K. Eds., Fitzpatrick's *Dermatology in General Medicine*, 8th ed., pp. 1147-1158. McGraw Hill Medical, NY.

The Coalition of Skin Diseases is the name of an umbrella association composed of member associations that provide education and support for people with specific skin diseases and disorders. Visit http://www .coalitionofskindiseases.org/ for information about the Coalition of Skin Diseases.

Listed below are other organizations that provide information and support for people with skin conditions.

Alopecia Areata
National Alopecia Areata Foundation
14 Mitchell Boulevard
San Rafael, CA 94903
Phone (415) 472-3780
E-mail info@naaf.org
www.naaf.org

Basal Cell Carcinoma Nevus Syndrome
Basal Cell Carcinoma Nevus Syndrome (BCCNS Life Support Network)
PO Box 321, 14525 North Cheshire Street
Burton, OH 44021
Phone (440) 834-0011
E-mail info@bccns.org
www.gorlinsyndrome.org, www.bccns.org

Cicatrical Alopecia
Cicatrical Alopecia Research Foundation (CARF)
9300 Wilshire Boulevard, Suite 410
Beverly Hills, CA 90212
Phone (310) 285-0525

E-mail info@carfintl.org
www.carfintl.org

Cutaneous Lymphoma
Cutaneous Lymphoma Foundation
PO Box 374
Birmingham, MI 48012
Phone (248) 644-9014
E-mail info@CLFoundation.org
www.CLFoundation.org

Ectodermal Dysplasias
National Foundation for Ectodermal Dysplasias (NFED)
6 Executive Drive, Suite 2
Fairview Heights, IL 62208-1360
Phone (618) 566-2020
E-mail info@nfed.org
www.nfed.org

Eczema
National Eczema Association
4460 Redwood Highway, Suite 16D
San Rafael, CA 94903
Phone (415) 499-3474
E-mail info@nationaleczema.org
www.nationaleczema.org

Epidermolysis Bullosa
Debra of America
16 East 41st Street, 3rd Floor
New York, NY 10017
Phone (212) 868-1573
E-mail staff@debra.org
www.debra.org

Ichthyosis
Foundation for Ichthyosis and Related Skin Types
2616 N. Broad Street
Colmar, PA 18915
Phone (215) 997-9400
E-mail info@firstskinfoundation.org
www.firstskinfoundation.org

Large Nevi and Related Disorders
Nevus Outreach, Inc.
600 SE Delaware, Suite 200
Bartlesville, OK 74003
Phone (918) 331-0595
www.nevus.org

Pachyonychia Congenita
Pachyonychia Congenita Project (PC Project)
2386 E. Heritage Way, Suite B
Salt Lake City, UT 84109
Phone (877) 628-7300
E-mail info@pachyonychia.org
www.pachyonychia.org

Pemphigus and Pemphigoid
International Pemphigus and Pemphigoid Foundation (IPPF)
1331 Garden Highway, Suite 100
Sacramento, CA 95833
Phone (916) 922-1298
E-mail info@pemphigus.org
www.pemphigus.org

Psoriasis
National Psoriasis Foundation
6600 SW 92nd Ave, Suite 300
Portland, OR 97219
Phone (503) 244-7404
E-mail getinfo@psoriasis.org
www.psoriasis.org

Sturge-Weber Syndrome and Klippel-Trenaunay
The Sturge-Weber Foundation
PO Box 418
Mt. Freedom, NJ 07970
Phone (973) 895-4445
E-mail swfl@sturge-weber.com
www.sturge-weber.org

Vitiligo
Vitiligo Support International, Inc. (VSI)
P.O. Box 3565

Lynchburg, VA 24503
Phone (434) 326-5380
E-mail info@vitiligosupport.org
www.vitiligosupport.org

Xeroderma Pigmentosum
Xeroderma Pigmentosum Family Support Group
8495 Folsom Boulevard #1
Sacramento, CA 95826
Phone (916) 379-0741
E-mail contact@xpfamilysupport.org
www.xpfamilysupport.org

INDEX

corticosteroids, topical, (cont.)
tis, 68; and Grover's disease, 87; and
lichen planus, 92; and lichen sclerosus,
86; and pityriasis lichenoides, 96; and
pityriasis rosea, 94
creatinine, 97
crotamiton, 71
cutaneous lymphomas, 124
cutaneous T-cell lymphoma (CTCL), 20,
49-55, 79, 96, 126, 127
cyclosporine, 41, 48, 59, 92, 126
cytokines, 34, 54, 55, 59, 76

dapsone, 59, 66, 127
denileukin difitox, 54
depression, 38, 98, 99, 101, 122
dermatitis, 38, 85; allergic, 82, 113;
contact, 82, 109, 113; frictional, 82;
seborrheic, 73, 81
dermatitis, atopic (AD, eczema), 33-41,
82, 117, 126; and anxiety and depression, 99; and aprepitant, 127; and capsaicin, 116; determination of, 96; itch
prevalence in, 15; and mediators and
receptors, 20; medications for, 111, 112,
113, 122, 123; and mu-opioid receptor
blockers, 125; and non-histaminergic
pathway, 18; parent's perspective on,
23-32; personal experience of, 3-12;
and phototherapy, 128; and pityriasis
rosea, 93; and pregnancy, 85; and
psychogenic itch, 98; and topical corticosteroids, 109; and water loss, 106;
and wet pajama treatments, 114; and
winter itch, 89
dermatitis herpetiformis, 63-66, 127
dermatographism (skin writing), 56, 57
dermatomyositis, 66-68, 126
desloratadine, 58, 119, 120
diabetes, 15, 79
dialysis, 75, 122, 124
dicloxacillin, 10
diphenhydramine, 58, 120, 121
doxepin, 113, 117, 123
drug-related itch, 96, 119

dry skin, 15, 34, 42, 72, 73, 78, 89, 105,
108, 111

eczema. *See* dermatitis, atopic (AD,
eczema)
eczema herpeticum, 10
emotions, 7-8, 38, 44, 50, 51. *See also*
anxiety; depression; stress
environment, 3, 6, 9, 29, 33, 38; and
climate/weather, 3, 6-7, 38, 58; and
humidity level, 7, 38, 39, 108. *See also*
temperature
epidermal growth factor receptor (EGFR)
inhibitors, 96, 127
epidermolysis bullosa congenita, 66
erythrocyte sedimentation rate (ESR), 97
etanercept, 48

fexofenadine, 58, 120, 121
fibromyalgia, 99
filaggrin, 34, 35
fluoxetine (Prozac), 124
fluvoxamine, 48, 123, 124
folliculitis, 71-72, 73
foods, 4, 8-9, 11, 19, 25, 26, 29, 38, 39,
56, 58

gabapentin, 48, 54, 61, 78, 122, 124
gastrin-releasing peptide receptor, 19
genes/heredity, 3, 11-12, 33, 34, 54
gluten intolerance, 63, 64
Gottron's sign, 67
G-protein coupled receptors, 18-19, 20
Grover's disease, 86, 87

hay fever, 33, 34
hematologic problems, 14, 123
hemodialysis, 15, 76, 78, 116
hepatitis C, 15, 78, 91
herpes, 82, 93
highly active antiretroviral therapy
(HAART), 73
histamine, 9, 18, 20, 40, 57, 58, 80, 117, 119
histamine receptors, 20, 57, 58
histone deacetylase (HDAC) inhibitors, 54